Francielle Vieira de Souza

Public Health Policies on American Tegumentary Leishmaniasis

Francielle Vieira de Souza

Public Health Policies on American Tegumentary Leishmaniasis

ScienciaScripts

Imprint

Cover image: www.ingimage.com

This book is a translation from the original published under ISBN 978-613-9-66823-6.

Publisher:
Sciencia Scripts
is a trademark of
Dodo Books Indian Ocean Ltd. and OmniScriptum S.R.L publishing group

120 High Road, East Finchley, London, N2 9ED, United Kingdom
Str. Armeneasca 28/1, office 1, Chisinau MD-2012, Republic of Moldova, Europe
Printed at: see last page
ISBN: 978-620-8-10985-1

SUMMARY

Summary

This study seeks to explore the links between health and the economy, specifically to describe the effects of different interventions on the control of American Tegumentary Leishmaniasis (ATL). Its general objective is to evaluate the effectiveness of policies to control ATL in the municipality of Montes Claros.

This is a qualitative, phenomenological, cross-sectional study, with a sample of 15 health professionals working in public hospitals, basic health units, zoonosis centres and epidemiological surveillance, who answered a semi-structured interview to find out their perceptions of ATL control policies. The data obtained was subjected to content analysis.

The following categories emerged from the analysis: knowledge about ATL and the priority given to the disease in the municipality, incidence and diagnosis of the disease, development of actions to control the disease, strategies related to the disease, decentralisation of services and resources earmarked for ATL control. The vast majority of interviewees believe that priority is given to ATL, that there has been an increase in the incidence of the disease, but are of the opinion that professionals do not know how to diagnose it. The interviewees were divided in their opinion about the development of control actions, with seven saying that they are not developed and seven saying that there are such actions, but the majority consider them to be unsatisfactory. There is no consensus on the decentralisation of control services and the vast majority of interviewees indicated that human and material resources are insufficient.

After analysing the results obtained, we can conclude that the disease is a health priority in most of the contexts under study, although there may be some cases of negligence in the fight against ATL. The officials interviewed have a correct perception of the evolution of the disease. It can be seen that in many cases ATL control measures are ineffective and in other cases no action is taken and the strategies used are limited to publicity actions. The decentralisation of control services has not been completed and human and material resources may be insufficient. In short, it can be concluded that there is no effectiveness in controlling ATL. In view of these conclusions, a set of suggestions has been put forward to improve the effectiveness of ATL control actions, which could improve the effectiveness of ATL control policies in the municipality of Montes Claros.

CHAPTER 1

INTRODUCTION

In the scientific field, health economics develops from systematic studies and research and the application of economic instruments as strategic and/or operational tools in the health sector. It is imperative to emphasise the important role of people's living conditions and their consequences on health when studying the dynamics of the health services market. Del Nero (2002) defines health economics as "the application of economic knowledge to the field of health sciences, in particular as a contributory element to the administration of health services" or, furthermore, a branch of knowledge whose objective is the optimisation of health actions, i.e. the study of the optimum conditions for the distribution of available resources to ensure the population the best possible health care and state of health, taking into account limited means and resources.

Health economics is currently a multidisciplinary field of scientific production and government action that is well developed in Europe, Canada, the United States and Australia, recognising that its knowledge is essential for those working in the planning, administration and management of health services. Despite the presence of international studies in the area dating back to the 1950s, it can be said that health economics has developed recently in Brazil. The creation of the Brazilian Association of Health Economics (ABRES) in 1989 can be taken as the basis for its establishment in the country. Since 1993, scientific production in the area has been institutionalised, mainly through support for international technical cooperation programmes between the UK and Brazil, coordinated by the Ministry of Health. Even so, there is a need for greater consolidation of this area in Brazil.

Saes (2000) considers the incorporation of health economics to be an indispensable aid in determining health management priorities, as it provides methodologies and/or management tools for economic evaluation, including studies of health supply and demand; studies relating to supplementary health and the organisation of service providers; evaluation of medical and diagnostic technologies; analysis of health systems, regulation and competition in this market and other possibilities (apud ANDRADE et al, 2007).

Health economic evaluation basically aims to answer two major questions: "Is the health strategy in question advantageous when compared to alternatives that could be implemented with these resources?" and "Are we aware and in agreement that the resources should be used in this way and not another?" (JUNIOR et *al,* 2011, p.1).

Health economics evaluates the relationship between the costs and effects of different interventions to determine the most efficient one, which offers the best return and allocation of resources (VIDAL et al, 2011).

Health policies in Brazil arose in the early twentieth century from economic strategies to clean up the agro-export corridors, and were initially consolidated around the control of endemic diseases.

The control of endemic diseases - which for several decades was the responsibility of the Foundation for Special Public Health Services (FSESP) and the Superintendence of Health Campaigns (SUCAM), now the National Health Foundation (FNS) - was initially carried out primarily in rural areas, through the actions of sanitary guards who, through police power, aimed to implement sanitary regulations and, through the use of technologies such as insecticides, eliminate the vectors that transmit these diseases (SILVA, 2001).

The pedagogical concepts that guided these actions - adjusted to the political and economic objectives in force - were archaic and uncritical. The individual was considered ignorant and devoid of any role in the production of knowledge, resulting in the establishment of unequal power and knowledge relations, impregnated with "cognitive arrogance" and devaluation of people's values and feelings. "This educational project weakened individuals, their self-esteem, their creative potential, their personal power to take initiatives and decisions, especially in the collective sphere" (OLIVEIRA, 2001, p.35).

According to Freese et *al* (1998 p.118), "the spread and persistence of certain epidemics and endemic diseases (schistosomiasis, cholera, malaria, leishmaniasis, dengue fever, etc.), for which treatment and technological solutions have been available for decades, militate against a definite transition process".

With this in mind, unlike the epidemiological transition that took place in the first world countries in the first half of the 20th century, when infectious and parasitic diseases were eradicated and/or controlled in parallel with the increase in chronic and degenerative diseases, "we are possibly facing a new *epidemiological pattern.* This is coupled with the still high rates of infectious and parasitic diseases (endemic/epidemic) and chronic and degenerative diseases, the so-called 'emerging and re-emerging' diseases, forming a highly complex and heterogeneous epidemiological profile, which presents unique characteristics and contradictions, when compared in the global/international context" (FREESE, 1998 p.109).

When we consider neglected diseases in the world, particularly in the Americas, we come across countless cases of diseases that have long since been eliminated in developed countries. Considering the parasitic and bacterial diseases identified as neglected worldwide, Hotez et *al.* (2007), include thirteen, among them three soil-transmitted verminoses (ascariasis, hookworm and trichuriasis), filariasis, onchocerciasis, dracunculiasis, schistosomiasis, Chagas disease, sleeping sickness, leishmaniasis, Buruli ulcer, leprosy and trachoma. An expanded list includes: dengue, treponematosis, leptospirosis, strongyloidosis, food-borne trematoidosis, neurocysticercosis, scabies, as well as "other tropical infections". This mention of the tropics, considered prejudiced and unscientific, is complemented by the statement that neglected diseases are "among the most common infections in a population estimated at 2.7 billion people living on less than US$ 2.0 a day" *(apud* CARVALHEIRO, 2008, p.03).

In the same vein, Hotez et *al.* (2008), based on prevalence and years of life lost (DALYs), consider that hookworm and other soil-transmitted verminoses, as well as Chagas disease, are the most important neglected tropical diseases in Latin America and the Caribbean. These diseases are followed by dengue, schistosomiasis, leishmaniasis, trachoma, leprosy and filariasis. In Brazil, the Department of Science and Technology of the Ministry of Health (Decit/MS) includes several of these diseases in its National Agenda of Health Research Priorities (BRASIL, 2006).

As a result, endemic diseases have once again been the focus of attention and have become a priority on the public policy agenda, due to the economic and social costs caused by their lack of control.

In recent decades, various movements, especially in Latin America and Brazil, have converged to consolidate new paradigms in the field of health that advance the understanding and approach to the health-disease process (SILVA, 2001).

Various fields of study already recognise the central role of health in conceptions of development, including its territorial dimension, which is particularly important for a country with the characteristics of Brazil. Recent theoretical contributions have brought to light the integration of health into the concept of development, as one of the determining factors of living conditions and well-being. The Human Development Index (HDI), which is the reference indicator most used in comparative analyses of the degree of development of national states, incorporates health as one of its three components. However, it would be an undesirable reductionism to restrict the relationship between health and development to this aspect of human capital, since there are several relationships between these fields (GADELHA et al, 2011).

According to Companhia Energética de Minas Gerais (CEMIG) (2006), the HDI was created by the United Nations (UN) in 1990 to be used as a more complete parameter than GDP in assessing the quality of life in all countries. In Brazil, studies carried out by the Institute of Applied Economic Research (IPEA), the Ministry of Planning and Budget, the João Pinheiro Foundation of the State of Minas Gerais and the Brazilian Institute of Geography and Statistics, in partnership with the United Nations Development Programme (UNDP), resulted in the creation of the Municipal Human Development Index (MHDI) and the Living Conditions Index (LCI). The M-HDI was created based on the same calculation methodology as the HDI, using income, life expectancy and education as a reference, but adapting these parameters to make them more representative of the Brazilian reality and adopting municipalities as the territorial units of analysis.

Vargas et al (2010) adds that the living conditions of the Brazilian population have improved significantly over the last few decades, as evidenced by the progressive increase in Brazil's average HDI in consecutive surveys. In 1960, Brazil's average HDI was 0.394, reaching 0.757 in 2000 and 0.813 in 2007.

Montes Claros' HDI-M is considered average by the UNDP. Its value is 0.783, the 101st highest in the entire state of Minas Gerais (out of 853 municipalities); 415th in the entire Southeast Region of Brazil (out of 1666) and 969th in the entire country (out of 5,507). The city has most of the average indicators, which are similar to the national average (UNDP, 2000).

According to Souza (2001), it is estimated that the number of poor people in Brazil represents approximately 30% of the total population, a proportion that is higher in the Northeast and North and in rural areas (39%), with poverty in the more industrialised states (mainly in the Southeast) being increasingly urban or, more predominantly, metropolitan.

In this context of social inequalities and scarcity of resources for health financing, evaluating the cost-benefit of actions and services is essential for drawing up strategies and programmes that respond to the real needs of the population. Although efficacy (the influence of technological innovations), effectiveness (the degree of approximation to possible improvements) and efficiency (cost savings without prejudice to goals) can be assessed, the use of health assessments should justify strategies and programmes and help rationalise public spending and the concept of efficiency (JUNIOR et *al,* 2011).

Particularly in the area of health, the Constitution and then Laws 8.080/90 and 8.142/901 set out the general guidelines for the organisation of a Unified Health System (SUS), which should provide more appropriate responses to Brazil's health problems. The trajectory of this system in the post-constitutional period has been quite tumultuous and criticised, particularly in terms of its ability to guarantee access and the quality of its services (MARQUES, 1999).

The proposals to reformulate the health care model, which were centred around the health reform movement, were instituted in 1988 by the Federal Constitution, with the creation of the SUS, based on an "important theoretical conceptual shift of the theme 'Health' from a strictly biological field to the political and historical field of the construction of rights" (BOSI, 1994, p.446).

Health is now considered a common good and a component of the exercise of citizenship and quality of life, "in the sense that each and everyone can be assured of exercising and practising this right to health, based on the application of all available wealth, knowledge and technology that society has developed and is developing in this field, appropriate to its needs, involving health promotion and protection; prevention, diagnosis, treatment and rehabilitation of diseases" (ALMEIDA et al, 2002, p.06).

Incorporating the paradigm of health promotion, the legislation defines the principles and guidelines of the SUS as universalisation, equity and comprehensive actions, as well as the political and managerial decentralisation of services, with a single directorate in each sphere of government and popular control of the system (BRASIL, 1995).

The Brazilian Constitution established that public health actions and services form part of a single command, organised in accordance with the guidelines of decentralisation, comprehensive care and community participation (Art. 198 of the Constitution). Its funding is made up of resources from the budgets of the federal, state and municipal governments, and social contributions, calculated on salaries, turnover and profit (Art. 195). The basic legal instruments regulating the implementation of the SUS were finalised at the end of 1990, with the publication of the Organic Health Law (8.080/90) and Law No. 8.142/90. The latter provides for community participation in the management of the SUS and intergovernmental transfers of financial resources.

It also adds the problem of its funding - lack of resources and a low degree of efficiency and effectiveness in its application, as well as difficulties in the relationship between the spheres of government and the private sector that provides services, jeopardising the results achieved and making the current situation of the SUS health care policy problematic. The deficiencies and distortions pointed out are recognised as strong enough to diagnose the unfeasibility of its model, which defines health care as universal, comprehensive and free, where access to any level of care depends on the user's initiative. There are various diagnoses that centre the discussion on the limitation of the SUS to the restrictions imposed by the federal government.

Although this level of government supported the creation of the system, it has shown contradictory behaviour to the development of the SUS in different administrations of the Ministry of Health, which today is still mainly responsible for conducting the decentralisation process in the area, since most of the financial resources come from it. The main obstacles to the issue have been the low priority given by the federal government to the area of health - not least because the nation's high public deficit imposes budgetary restrictions - and the failure to establish technical and transparent criteria for the distribution of all resources. Finally, some even recognise that the lack of resources is due to the fact that the care model continues to focus primarily on hospital care and not on basic health actions and services, including the most cost-effective actions (MARQUES, 1999).

From then on, the construction of new institutions and the production of services beyond the medical-hegemonic and bureaucratic-sanitary models have been a challenge for health managers and professionals (SILVA, 2001).

However, there is a growing perception that the health area is facing problems in its funding scheme, making it impossible to realise a more effective policy. In other words, with the deteriorating picture of health funding, plus the worsening of social issues in the country; deteriorating living conditions; unemployment; low wages; and concentration in income distribution, combined with the increase in population and the emergence of old diseases and new epidemics, further highlight the health crisis. As the health crisis has worsened, the agenda has narrowed until it is mainly focused on discussing the volume of financial resources from the federal government, characterised by a mere incrementalism in funding.

According to Marques (1999), it is important to emphasise the importance of building a new agenda that, without ignoring the generous principles of the SUS, considers that its implementation depends on a set of transformations, both managerial and in terms of care, as well as the solution of the country's macroeconomic problems.

As Medeiros (1999) points out, the scarcity of resources earmarked for health requires allocative decisions that consist of selecting the beneficiaries of the public health system and which services will be offered. The responsibility for these decisions, according to the author, is immense in a country like Brazil, where there is a great demand for health and where it is impossible for a large part of the population to obtain services outside the public system (apud ANDRADE et al, 2007).

Assis (2003) reinforces this thought when he says that we understand the need for efforts directed at daily struggles for a new model that prioritises health promotion, and that can also cope with the demand for care for illness with innovative social and institutional changes that reorient health policies and the organisation of services (public and private).

From this perspective, the Family Health Programme (PSF), which was originally based on various international experiences with similar aspects, was adopted by the Ministry of Health as a proposal to replace the current model of care.
This programme, characterised as a strategy that makes it possible to integrate and organise activities in a defined territory, aimed primarily at the family group, with a multidisciplinary and health promotion approach, has been progressively incorporated by various municipalities in the country, with specific characteristics based on the different local realities (SILVA, 2001).

With regard to endemic diseases, the legislation in force also transferred responsibility for planning, executing and managing control actions to the municipalities, with coordination at national, regional and state level. However, in the day-to-day running of services, the centralisation and verticalisation that has characterised endemic disease control programmes in Brazil for decades still prevails (FREESE, 1996).

The legislation moves forwards and backwards with regard to the decentralisation of health actions and services. It proposes mechanisms that aim to characterise the health responsibility of each manager, create a link between the citizen and the SUS, in short, mechanisms that make it possible to implement constitutional principles and guidelines, but effectively offers municipalities insufficient technical and financial support (SILVA, 2001).

Since decentralisation is a process that involves social, political, economic, ideological and cultural dimensions, local health managers are faced with a lack of organisational structure, financial resources, know-how that is coherent with users' needs, a lack of equal pay, power struggles between government bodies that have historically been responsible for certain jobs, in short, the obstacles that have characterised the reform of the Brazilian state.

The population, which in this new model is no longer just a user of the system but also responsible for it, has not been able to establish a dialogue with the services, occupy the formal spaces for participation and exercise social control. Thus, they find themselves dependent on a system that legally proposes to meet their health needs, but on the other hand, is often unable to meet even their need for reception (SILVA, 2001).

This includes the control and fight against American Tegumentary Leishmaniasis (ATL), which is the responsibility of the SUS and the municipalities, requiring human and material resources to be effective. The Ministry of Health, through its health service units, is responsible for preventing, treating and clarifying this infectious disease, which has a high incidence in South American countries such as Argentina. Bolivia, Chile, Peru and Brazil.

ATL is a zoonosis that affects both humans and various species of wild and domestic animals. Tonelli and Freire (2000) also conceptualise ATL as a disease caused by protozoa of the genus Leishmania, transmitted to humans by the bite of phlebotomines (Order Diptera; Family Psychodidae; Sub-Family Phlebotomina).

The World Health Organisation (WHO) estimates that 350 million people are at risk of acquiring the disease. The susceptibility or resistance of the vertebrate host to infection is related to the species of *Leishmania* and the host's immunological mechanisms (BOTELHO, 2006).

The worldwide incidence of leishmaniasis is two million cases, with 1 - 1.5 million new cases of tegumentary leishmaniasis (TL). TL is a serious health problem in Brazil, with 388,155 cases reported in the last 15 years (ALMEIDA & SANTOS,

2011).

Brazil is among the five countries that report more than 90 per cent of visceral leishmaniasis cases and among the seven with 90 per cent of tegumentary leishmaniasis cases worldwide. The urbanisation of leishmaniasis in the country is a public health problem and in recent decades outbreaks have occurred in several capital cities. The incidence of the disease has increased substantially and the under-recording of cases prevents us from knowing the magnitude of the problem (NUNES, 2006).

In recent years, the Ministry of Health has recorded an annual average of 35,000 new cases of ATL in the country. Minas Gerais reported 1922 cases of ATL in 2003. Between 2002 and 2010, the country recorded

The Municipal Health Department in the municipality of Montes Claros has treated 446 patients. At the moment, it is almost impossible to combat leishmaniasis using a single approach. A number of factors must be taken into account, such as vector control and antimonial therapy itself, the administration of which induces severe toxicity (BOTELHO, 2006).

With the growing number of reported cases, this disease became compulsorily notifiable from 1978 onwards and the ATL Control Programme has been successively structured. Actions related to vectors are the responsibility of the Superintendence of Endemic Disease Control (SUCEN); epidemiological investigation, diagnosis and treatment of cases are the responsibility of the Epidemiological Surveillance Centre (CVE), through the Regional Health Directorates (DIR), the State Health Department and the Basic Health Units (UBS) (GOMES & NEVES, 1998).

The ultimate goal of surveillance is the application of its product to disease prevention and control. Surveillance systems include the functional capacity to collect, analyse and disseminate information linked to public health programmes.

The knowledge produced by surveillance contributes to the continuous redefinition of public health priorities (CENTERS FOR DISEASE CONTROL, 1986).

The traditional zoonotic form reaches humans when they enter forest environments, where the natural foci of the disease are located. Therefore, human/forest contact is the primary determining factor in the occurrence of the disease. This epidemiological pattern predominated in the first decades of this century in the southeast and part of northeast Brazil. However, it still persists in areas of human occupation in the Amazon region. The increasing disappearance of forests has given rise to the phenomenon of the domiciliation of vectors, altering the condition in which humans are exposed to the parasite. The circulation of the causal agents in environments outside the geographical limits of the natural foci is increasing and induces the appearance of changes in the classic profiles of the disease. Another factor determining human exposure is demographic expansion, where the urbanisation process has been taking place close to the limits of natural foci, as well as in forest enclaves within cities (GOMES & NEVES, 1998).

Over the years, ATL has behaved as a classically occupational disease, typically affecting adult men exposed to forest regions. However, in recent decades it has shown changes in its epidemiological behaviour, given the extensive urbanisation process, with women and children increasingly being affected (MURBACK et *al,* 2011).

The city of Montes Claros, located in the north of the state of Minas Gerais, has an area of 101 km^2 , which corresponds to approximately 64% of the total area of the municipality and 94.22% of the municipal population, spatially poorly distributed, in which the peripheral neighbourhoods, especially those located to the east, north and south, are more densely occupied, due to a process of uneven and disordered urban expansion (LEITE et al, 2012).

The prospects for leishmaniasis vector control in a global strategy for the countries of the Americas will depend on a systematic review of the results of the programmes and the selective application of methods. Of course, the variety and epidemiological change in disease conditions must be taken into account, as well as the differences in infrastructure and basic resources with which the ATL control programme operates (GOMES & NEVES, 1998).

Its epidemiological importance is based on its prevalence and the different clinical pictures, which can evolve into severe and/or permanent mutilations. Oedemas, unsightly and invalidating infections, as well as affecting the individual's health, create a social problem by excluding the patient from the means of production that guarantee the family's livelihood and by the "stigma of the wound" that marks and segregates individuals from social interaction (SILVA, 2001, p.24).

This is based on considerations of the social importance given to the body and the implications of the leishmaniasis lesion for the carrier's body image and relationships. Costa et al (1987), in a study carried out in a Tegumentary Leishmaniasis endemic area in the interior of Bahia, found psychological and social disorders experienced by patients who had developed this disease in its severe form, ranging from relationship difficulties with the opposite sex to complete marginalisation by the community.

It is also a serious problem from an economic point of view, as the cost of implementing control programmes is high and often unsuccessful. One of the main factors contributing to this inefficiency is the fact that the leishmaniasis control programmes operated by the various local health systems were conceived within the same conceptual frameworks and strict logic that characterise endemic disease control programmes in Brazil.

These are not resolutive, partly because they do not recognise or fail to incorporate the network of social representations engendered in the daily lives of the populations affected into their approach to the health-disease process (SILVA, 2001).

Based on the analysis of the data on the new characteristic of the presentation of urbanisation of the disease, the municipal epidemiological profile of tegumentary leishmaniasis and the main risk factors that are associated with the appearance of cases of the disease (such as increased deforestation), it can be seen that the lack of efficient planning, aimed at more practical management of the disease, has been contributing negatively, favouring the appearance of epidemic outbreaks that compromise the health and quality of life of the population in the area studied.

This paper seeks to explore the links between health and the economy, based on the analytical premise that human beings have a right to health and subsidised by the public policy sphere. The importance of this analysis is particularised by the fact that a regional approach to designing policies for ATL has not yet been developed in the north of Minas Gerais. This has contributed to the increase in the number of cases of the disease, and we can already see that the concern of the relevant policies is only for Visceral Leishmaniasis, because it causes deaths quickly. However, the reality of the disease studied, like Visceral Leishmaniasis, produces devastating dermatological effects, and if left untreated, can evolve into the severe muco-cutaneous form and also cause death. The aim is to illustrate the complexity of these relationships by analysing the health services related to ATL in the Montes Claros macro-region.

The social and economic problems resulting from the lack of public policies aimed at solving environmental and health problems are of great importance. It is in this context that we primarily want to provide feedback to the Health Department of the Montes Claros region, with exploratory data on demand and the treatment sector, how and where the disease is publicised and a closer look at the relationship between management and tegumentary leishmaniasis. We want to pay attention to this dermatologically important disease, which has high rates of hospitalisation due to infection and even death, and which is unfortunately little studied by the relevant areas and thus also little known by the population. Economic evaluation studies of ATL are rare in the literature, and there is no study applied to the northern region of Minas Gerais.

It is in this context of concern that our study arises: To evaluate the effectiveness of the ATL control measures instituted in the Municipality of Montes Claros aimed at the population in its area of influence in 2012.

Specific objectives

- Characterise the municipality's human and financial resources involved in LTA control;

- To find out whether health service workers in the municipality of Montes Claros are aware of disease control policies;

- To describe the perception of health service workers in the municipality of Montes Claros about disease control measures, strategies used (including dissemination), level of commitment, treatment resources, level of decentralisation and effectiveness of the measures;

- To find out the opinion of health service workers in the municipality of Montes Claros on the care provided by health professionals and the supply of health facilities in relation to ATL;

- To compare the perception of the municipality's health service workers with the municipal statistics on the evolution of the disease;

- Characterise the ATL control actions carried out by the municipality's health services;

- Propose a set of guidelines for improving services.

The research is structured in five chapters: chapter one, now under analysis, presents general considerations about the chosen theme, the justifications that underpin its study and the general and specific objectives that it aims to achieve; chapter two presents the theoretical framework that supports the discussion of the data; chapter three is reserved for the presentation of the methodological procedures adopted for the collection, chapter four describes the treatment of the data, as well as its presentation and discussion in the light of the theoretical framework; finally, chapter five presents the final considerations.

CHAPTER 2

LITERATURE REVIEW

2.1. Health Policies in Brazil

In the early days of colonial Brazil and later in the Imperial phase, there was no organised state action on the health-disease process and the population fell victim to a wide variety of infectious diseases, making Brazil one of the unhealthiest countries on the planet (RONCALLI, 2000).

After the Proclamation of the Republic, health policies were established with a close link to Social Security, aimed at meeting political and economic interests, whether in the sanitation of economically important areas or in health care, with the aim of maintaining the individual as a productive workforce and with a type of organisation that favoured a process of privatisation through the purchase of care services, favouring the private sector (NÓBREGA et *al,* 2010).

At the end of the 1970s, the sector suffered from a lack of planning, discontinuity of programmes, cash flow problems, involvement in corruption schemes and misappropriation of funds, as well as inefficiency in services to meet the basic needs of the population (RONCALLI, 2000; OLIVEIRA & SOUZA, 1998).

The Health Reform Movement emerged at this time, led by health professionals and intellectuals from the field of collective health who, together with the population, were clamouring for more universalist policies. This movement was spreading its ideas and incorporating allies such as political union leaders, grassroots leaders, parliamentarians and even technicians from official health institutions. The milestone for this movement came in 1979, at the 1st National Symposium on Health Policies.

health. The Health Reform Movement, represented by the Centre for Brazilian Health Studies (CEBES (SUS)), presented and publicly discussed a new model for Brazil's health system, already called the Unified Health System (SUS), which would be rational, public, universal and decentralised (RONCALLI, 2000).

With the emergence of the SUS, there was a need to define objectives and strategic guidelines for the decentralisation process, as well as to standardise and operationalise relations between the spheres of government, dealing with aspects of responsibilities, relations between managers and criteria for transferring federal funds to states and municipalities. This led to the creation of the Basic Operational Standards (NOB) in 1991, one of the objectives of which was to establish criteria for the transfer of funds (BRASIL, 1991).

Then came NOB 93 and 96, the latter to implement automatic fund-to-fund transfers, creating the Basic Care Floor (PAB), a population-based payment modality that, over the years (1998 and 2000), was improved with the emergence of two types of PAB - fixed (per *capita/year)* and variable (resources for programmes defined by the federal level - such as the Community Health Agents Programmes (PACS) and the Family Health Programme (PSF), and the definition of guidelines for transferring resources to the PSF (NÓBREGA et al, 2010).

To help with the decentralisation process and to organise the health system at all levels, the Operational Standard for Health Care (NOAS) was published in 2001. The aim of this document was to generate decentralisation with autonomy, using financial resources according to real needs, as well as making clear the actions to prioritise basic procedures, with the creation of transfers such as the expanded PAB (BRASIL, 2001).

In its conception, the Brazilian SUS associates the territorial perspective with the decentralisation guideline, through the strategy of regionalising health actions and services. It is thus configured as a health system organisation project that must be unified, decentralised and hierarchical throughout the national territory, taking into account the country's regional diversity. This model has as its main objective the expansion of access to health (universality and comprehensiveness), attention to local needs, social participation and the efficient use of resources (GADELHA et al, 2011).

In the early years of implementing the SUS, this system was not supported by government policies and the resources needed to develop this process were not provided, aggravating the crisis of the care model that had been going on since the 1980s. As a result, the basic health network, made up of centres, clinics and basic health units (UBS), was disqualified and the next levels of care (secondary and tertiary) became the gateway to the system. The Family Health Programme (PSF) was created to reorganise healthcare practices on a new basis and replace the traditional model, bringing healthcare closer to families (BRASIL, 2001). The expansion of the PSF teams in Brazil and the organisation of the transfer of funds represent a significant advance in public health policies.

However, according to the ideas of Martinez & Martineau (2002), the organisation of health service management within the SUS remains an important problem to be solved, especially in the area of human resources, whose main challenges include precarious selection methods, low pay, poor team motivation, inequitable distribution of the workforce, low performance and unsatisfactory *accountability.*

According to the same author, other emerging challenges add to this situation, such as: the low qualifications and training of professionals to work with the health problems of communities, the aspect of human resource retention, which negatively affects the establishment of links, and the impact of epidemics on the health workforce - for example, the overload brought on by the H1N1 infection pandemic in several Brazilian cities, resulting in absenteeism, wear and tear and work overload.

According to Gadelha et al (2011), the health decentralisation strategy was not conceived in the context of a development model for the country. On the contrary, the development agenda left the national scene and was replaced by the debate on the re-democratisation of the state in the 80s and the search for currency stabilisation and control in the 90s. The hypothesis defended in the context of decentralisation was that the binomial reduction of the state and decentralisation of the management of public services would necessarily lead to an increase in the effectiveness of state action in the provision of essential goods and services to the population. In practice, however, decentralisation was essentially in line with the hegemonic and liberal trend, which contextualised the priority of downsizing the state and macroeconomic stabilisation.

In the day-to-day work of the PSF, it is common to find problems related to: (1) forms of contract; (2) material infrastructure (heterogeneity in the physical structure of family health units, some of which are inadequate and in a precarious situation); (3) the dynamics of care (overload of care that creates difficulties in planning and discussing the dynamics of work); and (4) the socio-political conditions for carrying out the work (different management styles of the family health teams, with relationships that are sometimes close and sometimes conflictual; these can also be highlighted; (5) contradictory expectations and conflicts between the family health teams and the local authorities; and (6) conflicts in the relationship between the PSF and the population, when the teams are unable to meet demand, for example (JUNQUEIRA et al, 2010).

The pace of implementation of this set of reforms has differed between countries, depending on the social protection model. In the Latin American region, reforms centred on the coordination of care are still in their infancy, which is reflected in the small number of studies dealing with this issue. The historical segmentation and fragmentation that has characterised most Latin American health systems, with selective primary health care, has weakened aspects such as the creation of integrated networks. Even so, in the context of the recent movement to value and defend the comprehensive concept of Primary Health Care, pro-coordination initiatives seem to be promising.

According to the authors, in these countries, although with varying degrees of development, the main strategies for integrating health systems are related to the territorialisation of services and client enrolment, computerisation of clinical histories, appointment centres, specialist teams as support for Primary Health Care, the creation of networks with regional and/or municipal management, among others (ALMEIDA et *al,* 2010).

With the aim of finding solutions to the precariousness of employment relationships in the three spheres of government, the Ministry of Health has created the National Programme for the Depayment of Work in the SUS (Desprecariza SUS). This initiative takes into account the size and needs of the states and municipalities. Among the intervention proposals are actions aimed at sensitising and making managers aware of the need to draw up and implement a new human resources policy (JUNQUEIRA et *al,* 2010).

However, according to Nogueira (2006), the expression "job insecurity" can give the false idea that workers who have benefited from a policy to repair the lack of respect for their rights will be kept in the job they have been doing. However, those who are already "precarious", because they are irregular, will sooner or later have to leave their jobs, to be replaced by regular workers who will join the public administration through public tenders. Therefore, what is at stake is the implementation of a situation of legality of employment relationships, and the best name that can be given to such a policy would be the regularisation of employment relationships.

The Brazilian experience reveals the complexity of health in an immense, unequal country, with a federative political system, which is continually strained by various structural and conjunctural obstacles. In turn, the analysis of the decentralisation of health reflects the contradictions and impasses in the construction of the regional approach of this policy, which has as its central issue the organisation of actions and services in the territory (GADELHA et al, 2011).

With a total of 5,564 municipalities, the majority of Brazil today is made up of small municipalities, with 4,075 municipalities (73.1%) having a population of up to 20,000 inhabitants. This data establishes small municipalities as one of the main protagonists in the implementation and management of the SUS, and they cannot be left off the list of priorities (CONASEMS, 2007).

According to Gadelha et al (2011), the role of the states was stripped away, making it difficult, or even impossible in some cases, to coordinate and plan the entire system based on a territorial logic. The process of municipalisation, on the one hand, allowed for the establishment of the SUS by expanding access to healthcare, but on the other, it led to the creation of thousands of "isolated local systems". Local governments assumed responsibility for the provision of health services, in a context where most municipalities had a small population base and limited institutional capacity, which hampered the regional planning function.

We will now give an overview of the organisation of the health system in the state of Minas Gerais and the municipality of Montes Claros, where this study was carried out.

The state of Minas Gerais is divided into 13 health macro-regions, which are made up of 75 micro-regions, according to the Regionalisation Master Plan. The macro-region under study is the North of Southeast, made up of 89 municipalities and divided into seven health micro-regions: Bocaiúva (5 municipalities), Grão Mongol (6 municipalities), Janaúba (12 municipalities), Januária (16 municipalities), Montes Claros (22 municipalities), Pirapora (10 municipalities) and Salinas (17 municipalities).

The macro-region under study has a total population of 366,134 inhabitants and a total of 8,780 health professionals, which gives a ratio of approximately 45 inhabitants for each health professional.

In the public sector, the municipality has thirteen basic health units, classified as Montes Claros Health Centres, and six general hospitals, one public, two private and three philanthropic.

Coordination between levels of care can be defined as the articulation between the various health services and actions related to a given intervention so that, regardless of where they are provided, they are synchronised and aimed at achieving a common goal. In this sense, it is reflected in the existence of an integrated network, from Primary Health Care to the most technologically dense providers, so that different care interventions are perceived and experienced by the user in a continuous manner, appropriate to their health care needs and compatible with their personal expectations. Therefore, care coordination would be an organisational attribute of health services that translates into the perception of continuity of care from the user's perspective (ALMEIDA et *al,* 2010).

In Brazil, the reorganisation of actions at local level has not been homogeneous. Firstly, due to the small size of many municipalities, which faced difficulties in planning and organising their systems; secondly, due to the uneven distribution of human resources and installed capacity and, finally, due to the characteristics of municipal governments and the management of local systems (CUNHA & SILVA, 2010).

An investigation carried out by Escorel et *al.* (2007) in ten state capitals with PSFs in place revealed the existence of access barriers due to inadequate opening hours and difficulties in meeting spontaneous demand. A case study carried out in five municipalities in the state of Bahia analysing the decentralisation of management revealed that there had been an increase in healthcare coverage in all the municipalities analysed. However, access to services encountered barriers both in primary care and in medium and high complexity care. Other studies dealing with this issue focus on describing the characteristics of service use or estimates of service coverage related to the expansion of service provision, as well as evaluating some variables in the organisation of services as components of accessibility.

2.2. Organisation of the Brazilian health system and distribution of financial

resources: the quest for decentralisation and management autonomy

Discussions and problems linked to the coordination of health care, the fragmentation of the care network and the lack of communication between providers are not new topics in discussions about the organisation of health systems. However, recent changes in relation to the demands and needs of the population with the growing prevalence of chronic diseases, which require greater contact with health services in a context of pressure to optimise cost-efficiency ratios, have made the search for solutions urgent. In the European Union, pro-coordination reforms have been implemented since the 1990s, mainly aimed at strengthening the first level of care (ALMEIDA et *al,* 2010).

Federal spending over the years has followed an upward trend, which is interesting when you consider the political and economic context of the time (financial paralysis in Latin America, the need for a larger primary surplus, small amounts *per capita* earmarked for health). These gains in health investments increased considerably with the issue of decentralisation, accompanied by the inclusion of municipalities in responsibility for services by directing and increasing their resources in the sector. As a result, there was also an increase in investments to enable municipalities to set up management systems.

The search for an organised decentralisation process can be found in various official documents such as the SUS Basic Operational Standard (NOB-96), the Integrated Agreed Programming (PPI - 1997) and the Health Care Operational Standard (NOAS -2001). NOB 96 defines important principles such as a set of responsibilities and requirements for municipalities to qualify for a type of management, where the decision on this process was left to the bipartite inter-management committees (municipality and state-CIB). Thus, in December 1998, 4,597 municipalities were qualified for Full Primary Care Management (equivalent to 83%); in 2000, 99% of municipalities were already qualified for this type of management.

Decentralisation, municipalisation and incentives for qualification are important because they decentralise and organise health resources, thus reaching thousands of municipalities that, until then, did not receive transfers from the federal level and had no management autonomy (NÓBREGA et *al,* 2010).

An important fact regarding the collection of funds for health was Law No. 9,311 of 24 October 1996, which created the Provisional Contribution on Financial Transactions (CPMF) (BRASIL, 1996).

Projections of resources for the health sector made in 1995 for the following year indicated that the system would collapse, so alternatives were sought and, after extensive political debate, the CPMF Law was passed. Initially, the contribution was set at 0.20 per cent on financial transactions, with a defined duration of thirteen months (NÓBREGA et al, 2010).

The funds were transferred directly to the National Health Fund (FNS), totalling R$6.9 billion in 1997. In the following years, as the federal budget was already dependent on these resources, the CPMF was extended for a further 36 months, with a rate of 0.38%, of which 0.20% was for health and 0.18% for social security. The great controversy surrounding the CPMF was that the federal government used health as a pretext for approving the "tax" and, according to the law, would transfer the funds directly to the National Health Fund (FNS), but in return stopped passing on other funds that were previously earmarked for health. The CPMF was a decoy, because the federal government earmarked this revenue for health, but in return stopped passing on revenue from other sources, leaving the final result of the health budget almost unchanged: "it gave with one hand and took away with the other" (CARVALHO, 2002, p.245).

Data from the Social Studies Directorate of the Institute for Applied Economic Research (IPEA) shows that health funding from contributions such as the Social Contribution for the Financing of Social Security (COFINS) fell by around 4% between 1997 and 1999. CPMF funds increased by around 21 per cent between

1997 and 1998 alone; on the other hand, the amounts in 1999 were already 24 per cent lower than the same funds collected in the previous yearAnother factor contributing to the issue of the distribution of financial resources in the public sector is Constitutional Amendment 29, which has been a legal and fundamental point since 2000.

This amendment establishes an increase in investment by the three government sectors (federal, state and municipal) in the health sector, thus guaranteeing minimum resources for health actions and services and even prohibiting the use of funds earmarked for health to pay for inactive workers. The amendment altered article 34 of the Federal Constitution, including a minimum requirement of state tax revenue, as well as extending the Union's power to intervene in the states if they fail to fulfil their obligation to allocate the established percentage of revenue. The percentage that each municipality must spend on health is also included in the amendment; from 2000, when it was instituted, to 2004, this minimum percentage increased from 7% to 15%.

This process of participatory management is important for the whole area of health and has been demonstrated in numbers and figures: in 2000, 5,450 municipalities were already receiving fund-to-fund transfers, which is equivalent to 61 per cent of federal resources for health costs. That same year, specific amounts were implemented for full management, which in five years went from around eleven thousand reais (in 2000) to a total of approximately 5.5 billion reais in 2006. This management autonomy is incentivised by additional transfers that increase every year as a way of encouraging it to cover a larger number of municipalities.

According to data from the Institute for Applied Economic Research (IPEA), during then President Fernando Henrique Cardoso's first term in office (1995-1998), spending on health programmes decreased over the years. In millions of reais, the figure went from 17,774 in 1995 to 14,038 in 1998, showing a negative variation in investments of around 21 per cent. According to the PAHO-WHO report, federal spending by the Ministry of Health in 1996 was 10.4 per cent of the Union's revenue, a figure lower than health spending in 1989, which was around 19 per cent (NÓBREGA et *al,* 2010).

This was one of the factors that encouraged Health Minister Adib Jatene at the time to fight for another source of funds for health financing, thus creating the CPMF. During Fernando Henrique Cardoso's (FHC) second term in office, the economist

José Serra took over the Ministry of Health, obtaining more sources of funding with the approval of Constitutional Amendment 29 and the creation of the PAB (BRASIL, 1997).

Financing the SUS is a joint responsibility of the three levels of government. In September 2000, Constitutional Amendment 29 (EC-29) was approved, which determined that revenues from all three levels should be earmarked for the system. Federal funds, which account for more than 70% of the total, have progressively been passed on to states and municipalities through direct transfers from the National Health Fund to state and municipal funds, in accordance with the mechanism established by decree 1,232 of 30 August 1994. The intense qualification of municipalities and states in advanced management modalities led to a significant increase in direct transfers of resources from the National Health Fund to municipal and state funds, so that by December 2001, most of the assistance resources were already transferred in this modality, as opposed to the predominance of direct federal payment to service providers. In addition to transfers from the National Health Fund, state and municipal funds receive contributions from their own budgets. Some states transfer their own resources to municipal health funds, according to rules defined at state level. The federal level is still responsible for the largest share of SUS funding, although the participation of municipalities has been growing over the last ten years and there is a prospect that the share of state resources in funding the system will increase significantly

as a result of the approval of EC-29 (MARQUES, 1999).
However, despite the efforts to organise health in Brazil during the FHC period, vital reforms and fiscal adjustments to achieve macroeconomic stability put health and social policies on the back burner, which may partly explain the differences in the amounts allocated to health from the federal budget in the different governments. The issue of focussing health policies in this period is very clear, with the deliberation of medical and hospital care and the emergence of the private segment as supplementary health for the population that has an income that makes these services possible. This supplementary health policy is a historical issue that did not begin during this period and remains active to this day (COSTA, 2002).

The indemnification of funding sources for health, enshrined in the Constitution, led to the need for a constitutional amendment. Although Constitutional Amendment 29 rescued the percentage allocation of resources for health in the three spheres of government (a minimum of 15% of own revenues for municipalities, a minimum of 12% for states and a nominal variation in GDP for the Union), it remains pending regulation by ordinary law. Meanwhile, municipalities, states and the federal government, taking advantage of interpretations by the Courts of Auditors, have been allocating lower percentages that are incompatible with the needs of the SUS system (BORGES, 2009).

Despite the political and economic problems in our country, the organisation of healthcare began to show results in the second FHC administration, and continued to receive inputs and additions during the first administration of Luiz Inácio Lula da Silva (2002-2005). This is due to the maintenance and expansion of FHC administration programmes, as well as the creation of new DATASUS programmes (NÓBREGA et al, 2010).

2.3. Unifying pacts and equity

One of the reasons for believing in a restructuring of the Brazilian Health System is the creation of the Pact for Health. The Pact for Health is a set of institutional reforms of the SUS, defined in Ministerial Order GM No. 399 of 22 February 2006, agreed between the three spheres of management (Union, states and municipalities), with the aim of promoting innovations in management processes and instruments, in order to achieve greater efficiency and quality in the responses of the Unified Health System. At the same time, the Pact for Health redefines the responsibilities of each manager according to the health needs of the population and in the pursuit of social equity (BRASIL, 2006).

The 2006 Pact for Health established the freedom to adapt strategies to different realities, making it possible to create new centralities and new management arrangements in the organisation of the healthcare model. In this context, there has been a change in the definition of region, with the proposal of different designs for health regions (understood as sections of intra-municipal, intra-state, inter-state and border geographical spaces), implying recognition of specificities and the agreed political-institutional arrangement. Also in the context of the Pact, it is assumed that the region must meet criteria that provide resolution to the territory, with sufficiency in basic care and part of medium complexity (GADELHA et al, 2011).

The ways in which federal funds are transferred to states and municipalities were also modified by the Pact for Health, and are now integrated into five major funding blocks (Primary Care, Medium and High Complexity Care, Health Surveillance, Pharmaceutical Care and SUS Management), thus replacing the more than one hundred "little boxes" that were used for this purpose (NÓBREGA et *al,* 2010).

The proposal for primary health care, expressed at the Alma-Ata Conference, represented a conceptual and technological innovation in the vision of health systems around the world, by defending the principles of comprehensiveness, quality, equity and social participation in health. These principles would be achieved through a decentralised network of health services, capable of accommodating and resolving most of the health problems of individuals and communities, prioritising the most vulnerable social groups (WHO, 1978).

This pact presents significant changes for the implementation of the SUS, including the replacement of the current qualification process with joint adherence to management commitment terms; joint and cooperative regionalisation as the structuring axis of the decentralisation process; the integration of the various forms of transfer of federal funds and the unification of the various pacts that currently exist. It is the result of an intense two-year discussion involving technicians and management from the various areas of the Ministry of Health, the National Council of Municipal Health Secretaries (CONASEMS) and the National Council of Health Secretaries (CONASS), and was approved at the Tripartite Interagency Commission meeting on 26 January 2006 and at the National Health Council meeting on 9 February 2006 (NÓBREGA et al, 2010).

The implementation of this pact, in its three dimensions - Pact for Life, in Defence of the SUS and for Management - makes it possible to implement agreements between the three spheres of SUS management to reform current institutional aspects, promoting innovations in management processes and instruments aimed at achieving greater effectiveness, efficiency and quality in their responses and, at the same time, redefining collective responsibilities for health results according to the population's health needs and in the pursuit of social equity (BRASIL, 2006).

The implementation of the SUS in the early 1990s was of fundamental importance in guaranteeing and expanding the population's access to health services. To this end, the decentralisation of management was strategically induced by the formulation and establishment of operational and health care standards, issued between 1993 and 2002, which sought to consolidate the full exercise of municipal public power in the role of health care manager. More recently, the health pact proposed new guidelines for health policies, reaffirming municipalisation and the organisation of the system through primary care as the way to consolidate the SUS (CUNHA & SILVA, 2010).

Since 1994, with the progressive implementation of the Family Health Strategy, basic health care in Brazil has been strengthened, anchored in the principles of comprehensive and hierarchical care, territorialisation, population registration and multi-professional teams.

Reinforced by the growth in coverage of the Family Health Strategy and the prominence it received in the latest World Health Report, primary care could be qualified by updating information on the demand it meets, so as to enable it to make an effective contribution to the management of the health system (TOMASI et al, 2011).

However, even though the territorial issue has been given a new treatment in the Pact for Health, implicit in these guidelines is a concept of regionalisation that still carries with it two basic assumptions: (1) that of guaranteeing access to health services, seeking to address different situations with a better and quicker response to users' wishes and needs; and (2) that of the rational deployment of health resources, which should be organised according to a hierarchical logic, with the aim of optimising spending based on efficiency gains resulting from combining the advantages of local provision with economies of scale in the actions and services provided. A slightly closer look allows us to consider that the Pact's assumptions will not be able to advance substantially without a new renegotiation of the criteria for transferring resources; without considering the regional logic that needs to be planned and agreed between the three spheres of government, with a recovery of the role of the federated units in this process; and without a greater contribution of resources that responds to the necessary deconcentration of the infrastructure of health goods and services (GADELHA et al, 2011).

The same author states that there is still a balance to be struck between decentralising health services and concentrating them at intermediate, micro or mesoregional levels, as well as at central, macro-regional or national levels. The presence of multiple scales requires that the debate on a regional policy be able to articulate the territorialisation of actions with the specificities of each field of health activity and its internal logics, as well as the flows and organisation of spaces. In other words, it requires a maturing of the articulation of actors, effective coordination and an increase in the contribution of resources.

Borges (2009) states that unlike universalisation, comprehensiveness is a challenge that can be overcome. It allows for rationality, as long as it is scientifically supported. The SUS should guarantee Brazilians the comprehensive care necessary for a healthy life, including prevention, promotion and treatment. However, there is a reasonable consensus in our society that the right to comprehensive care should be based on scientific evidence and ethical principles that are socially validated. This makes it possible to organise provision within rational and truly health-impacting standards. The Ministry of Health has endeavoured, together with states and municipalities, to negotiate evidence-based protocols to regulate the supply of SUS services, submitting them to the Health Councils. A permanent assessment of new technological additions, whether in the area of medicines or diagnostic and therapeutic equipment, is necessary. Regulated integrality is needed in the SUS, as Gilson Carvalho advocated during his time at the Ministry of Health (Health Care Secretariat - SAS).

2.4. Health Services Management

Health service management is an administrative practice that aims to optimise the way organisations work in order to achieve maximum efficiency (the relationship between products and resources employed), effectiveness (achieving the objectives set) and effectiveness (solving the problems identified). In this process, the manager uses knowledge, techniques and procedures that enable him or her to steer the operation of services in the direction of the defined objectives.

One obstacle to the wider use of evaluation in decision-making in health services is that its implementation requires resources and time, which makes it difficult to use it for problems that need immediate solutions. In these situations, which are frequent when it comes to the health of people and the population, only the existence of accumulated knowledge, resulting from past or previously planned evaluations, can contribute to decision-making (TANAKA and TAMAKI, 2012).

Evaluation is an essential management support tool because of its ability to improve the quality of decision-making. Despite this, its use is still incipient in the management of health services (VAUGHAN, 1999).

Evaluation can be referred to as knowledge produced in the theoretical-methodological field applicable to an object when there is a need to make a value judgement, regardless of the use that will be made of its product. This conception of evaluation creates its own field of knowledge for evaluation, increasing its interface with the field of research (HARTZ, 1997).

Management involves improving the way organisations work and to do this it has to find the best possible combination of available resources to achieve its objectives. Once this combination has been found, it is institutionalised through the formalisation of structures, processes, routines, flows and procedures.

All this construction is designed to achieve optimal functioning in a complex context, characterised by the set of factors that condition health and illness and which constantly produce unpredictable situations that require decision-making. There is a need to respond to these situations in order to maintain the functioning or improve the levels of efficiency and effectiveness of the services (TANAKA and TAMAKI, 2012).

Decision-making in health management is complex and permeated with subjectivity and uncertainty. Paim and Teixeira (2006, p.76-78), referring to the area of health policies, planning and management, emphasise these characteristics by stating that: "there are *times when there is a lack of knowledge for decision-making, others when there is sufficient knowledge but decisions are postponed, and still others when decisions are necessary even in the face of scant evidence"*.

Providing managers with timely information is essential for improving the quality of decisions. If there is accumulated knowledge from past research, studies and evaluations, the appropriate procedure consists of appropriating this knowledge and using it in the decision-making process. If not, it is necessary to structure an evaluation process that is as consistent as possible within the time and resources available.

In the routine of health services, the need to solve the population's health problems or satisfy user demands limits the time for decision-making, as it is necessary to respond to situations that are already being experienced by the manager. This means that evaluations tend: to be carried out quickly; to use information and knowledge that is already available; to use methodological tools that suit the time and resources available; to reduce and simplify the elements to be studied; and to use a degree of precision (level of confidence) in the results that is sufficient for the decision to be made (TANAKA and TAMAKI, 2012).

According to the World Health Organisation (1981), the choice of an indicator must take into account its validity (effectively measuring what it is intended to measure), its reliability (presenting the same result even if it is used by different people or in different circumstances), its sensitivity (ability to capture changes in the situation or object being studied), and its specificity (reflecting changes only in the object being studied).

As mentioned by the Inter-Agency Network on Health Information (2002), depending on the application of the indicators, other attributes can be added to these: measurability (based on data that is available or easy to obtain); relevance (responding to health priorities); and cost-effectiveness (the results justify the investment of time and resources).

Decision-making is a responsibility and a formal competence of the manager who, in addition to the information obtained in the evaluation process, uses the personal knowledge they have (technical references, institutional policies, social, cultural and others) or their perception of the problem, forms a conviction and makes a decision, mobilising the necessary resources (TANAKA and TAMAKI, 2012).

It is in this context that we are studying this subject, with a view to researching LTA control programmes, which we will address next.

2.5. American Tegumentary Leishmaniasis: control issues We will now describe the epidemiological aspects of ATL and its control.

2.5.1. Epidemiology of the disease

It should be noted that health research shows that the worst health indices are found among the most vulnerable population groups located at the bottom of the social pyramid. These disparities can be seen in living and health conditions between different social groups and between different geographical areas of the same country. Epidemiology has traditionally dealt with this issue, and countless studies point to the inequalities in getting sick and dying in society, highlighting the differences in relation to place, time, age and sex, as well as between groups, ethnicities, gender and social classes (VIANA et al, 2003).

ATL is an infectious disease of the skin and mucous membranes, the etiological agent of which is a protozoan of the Leishmania genus (PENNA et al, 2011).

Because it has different clinical and epidemiological characteristics in each geographical area, leishmaniasis is described in four groups: Cutaneous leishmaniasis, which produces skin lesions, ulcerative or not; cutaneous-mucosal or mucocutaneous leishmaniasis, a form that is complicated by the appearance of destructive lesions on the mucous membranes of the nose, mouth and pharynx; visceral leishmaniasis or kala-azar, in which the parasites show a marked tropism for the spleen, liver, bone marrow and lymphoid tissues; and diffuse cutaneous leishmaniasis, a disseminated form that appears in anergic individuals or, later, in patients who had been treated for kala-azar (REY, 1991, p. 182).182). ATL includes cutaneous leishmaniasis (CL) and mucosal leishmaniasis (ML).

According to Gontijo and Carvalho (2003 p.74) "mucosal leishmaniasis, also known as sputa, is difficult to treat and has a poor prognosis in terms of the possibility of a cure. It is associated with L. braziliensis, in most cases occurring within a variable period of time after the initial skin lesion has appeared. The factors that contribute to an initially cutaneous disease evolving into this late form are not entirely known, but it is known that delayed healing of the primary lesion and inadequate initial treatment may be associated" (Figure 1-B).

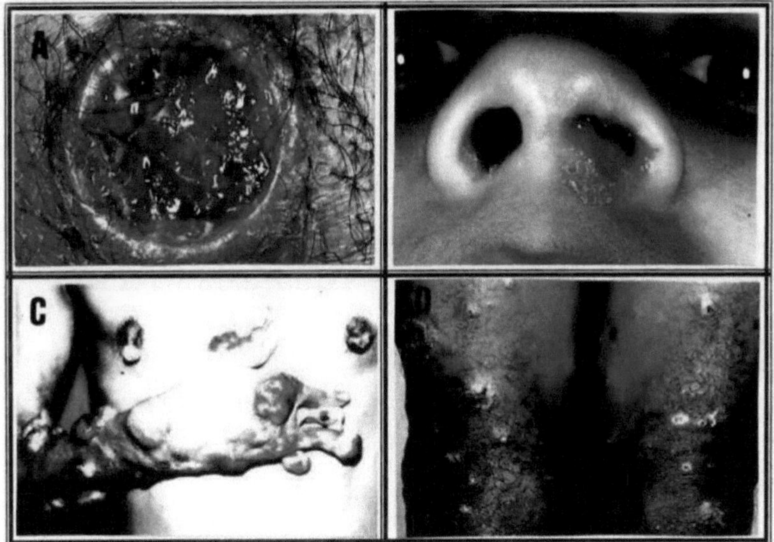

Figure 01- ATL: (A) Cutaneous form (classic frame lesion); (B) Mucosal form; (C) Diffuse form; (D) Disseminated form.

Source: GONTIJO & CARVALHO, 2003.

Mucosal involvement can appear while the skin lesion is still active, or years after it has healed. Among the mucosal lesions, the following varieties can be distinguished: ulcer-infiltrating, polyposis and terebrant. In almost all cases, ML affects the nasal mucosa, with significant involvement of the septum, followed in order of frequency by involvement of the oral mucosa. In both cases, the risk of permanent deformities is considerable. The involvement of mucous membranes other than those of the upper airways is exceptional (GONTIJO; CARVALHO, 2003).

Even in a small percentage of patients with ML or mucocutaneous lesions, they are a particularly important manifestation due to the deforming sequelae with anatomical, psychological and social acceptance consequences, which alter the patient's quality of life and can lead to death as a result of complications.

It is characterised by metastatic spread to the mucous membranes, secondary to cutaneous leishmaniasis, mainly nasal, although the literature records it as rare in other mucous membranes, such as the genital and ocular (TONELLI & FREIRE, 2000).

Among the less common forms of ATL is diffuse cutaneous leishmaniasis (DCL) (Figure 1-C), located in the anergic pole of the disease, as opposed to the resistant polar form represented by mucosal cutaneous leishmaniasis (MCL) and part of localised cutaneous leishmaniasis (LCL) (GONTIJO ; CARVALHO, 2003).

The WHO reports the occurrence of leishmaniasis in 88 countries, with compulsory notification in only 32 and an estimated 12 million people affected by the disease in Asia, Africa, Europe and the Americas. Approximately 350 million people live in areas of transmission and it is estimated that there are two million new cases a year, of which 1.5 million are cutaneous and cutaneomucosal and 500,000 visceral.

ATL occurs in the Americas from the south of the United States to the north of Argentina. The most important focus is South America, which includes all countries except Uruguay and Chile. The incidence of the disease in Brazil has increased over the last 20 years, with cases recorded in all states, affecting people of all age groups and both sexes. Epidemic outbreaks have occurred in the Southeast, Midwest, Northeast and, more recently, in the Amazon region, due to the predatory colonisation process. Between 1980 and 2003, the Ministry of Health recorded an annual average of 23,000 cases of ATL in Brazil (LIMA et al, 2007).

From the 1980s onwards, there was a significant increase in the number of registered cases: from 3,000 in 1980 to 37,710 cases in 2001. Transmission peaks have been observed every five years and, from 1985 onwards, there has been an upward trend in the number of cases (BRASIL, 2007).

In the 1990s, the Ministry of Health reported an annual average of 32,000 new cases of ATL. Analysing the data for 2003, the situation was as follows: the Northern Region reported approximately 45% of cases, predominantly in the states of Pará, Amazonas and Rondônia; the Northeastern Region, 26% of cases, mainly in Maranhão, Bahia and Ceará; the Central-Western Region, 15% of cases, most frequently in the state of Mato Grosso; the Southeastern Region, 11% of cases, predominantly in Minas Gerais; and the Southern Region, 3.0%, with Paraná standing out (BRASIL, 2006).

Between 1999 and 2008, 269,122 cases of ATL were recorded, with an annual average of 26,912 cases. The disease occurs predominantly in adult males, although recently a greater involvement of children of both sexes has been documented (PENNA et al, 2011).

In the state of Minas Gerais (MG), ATL has occurred since the middle of the century with outbreaks related to deforestation and the construction of motorways, as well as the development of agriculture (FURTADO et *al.,* 1966).

Currently, in the state of Minas Gerais, ATL is present in practically every municipality, in areas where roads and hydroelectric dams have been built and where groups of people have settled. As well as its continued presence in former endemic hotspots of the Atlantic Forest and in the Rio Doce and Mucuri valleys, numerous cases have also been reported in urban areas of large and medium-sized cities, such as Belo Horizonte, Montes Claros and Governador Valadares (BARATA et al, 2011).

In the context of public health, ATL has grown significantly in importance due to the growing process of urbanisation. Initially, the disease was eminently rural in nature and, more recently, it has been spreading to medium and large urban areas, as is the case in the municipality of Montes Claros (Chart 1).

Chart 1- Distribution of patients with American tegumentary leishmaniasis according to area of residence in the municipality of Montes Claros from 2002 to 2010

Variable	Number of cases (n=446)	%
Area of residence		
Urban	342	76,68
Countryside	92	20,63
Urban/Rural	3	0,67
Ignored	9	2,02

Source: Montes Claros City Hall, 2010

2.5.2. Clinical manifestations

The condition is usually asymptomatic, predominantly in uncovered areas of the body and develops in patients from endemic areas or who have been there recently. It can have an abortive course or take on a torpid character, ending in spontaneous regression, as observed in several Brazilian foci. In most cases, the infection progresses and, after a period of clinical latency lasting several months, skin and/or mucous membrane lesions appear as a result of the parasite's haematogenous and/or lymphatic dissemination (FURTADO, 1994).

Cutaneous leishmaniasis (CL) is defined by the presence of lesions exclusively on the skin, which begin at the point of inoculation of infective promastigotes, through the bite of the vector, for any of the species of Leishmania that cause the disease. The primary lesion is usually a single one, although multiple phlebotomine bites or local dissemination can generate a large number of lesions (MARZOCHI, 1992).

It appears after a variable incubation period of 10 days to three months, as an erythematous papule that slowly progresses to a nodule. It is accompanied by regional adenopathy, with or without lymphangitis, in 12 to 30 per cent of cases. As it progresses, the notable polymorphism of the lesions is emphasised and it is possible to find impetigoid, lichenoid, tuberculous or lupoid, nodular, vegetating and ectimatoid forms. Ulcerations with raised, indurated borders and a background of coarse granulation tissue are frequent, configuring the classic lesion with a framed border (GONTIJO & CARVALHO, 2003) (Figure 1-A).

The most frequent location of the lesions on the body is in the areas exposed to the transmitter's bites, mainly on the lower limbs, feet, followed by the upper limbs, face, neck, chest, auricular pavilions, penis, etc. Sometimes leishmaniotic ulcers can take on atypical aspects that are difficult to diagnose. Approximately 75% of patients in Leishmania brasiliensis areas in Brazil have a single lesion (TONELLI & FREIRE, 2000).

In Brazil, ATL is an important public health problem due to the growing number of human cases. The infection can cause mutilating lesions and lead to loss of ability to work and even death.

2.5.3. Etiology and transmission mechanisms

ATL is a disease caused by protozoa of the genus Leishmania, transmitted to humans by the bite of phlebotomines (Order Diptera; Family Psychodidae; Sub-Family Phlebotomina) (TONELLI & FREIRE, 2000).

The great epidemiological importance of leishmaniasis is the driving force behind studies of phlebotomines, which are the vectors of *Leishmania.* More than 800 species of these insects have been described and it is estimated that 81 of them are capable of transmitting these parasites. Phlebotomines also have vectorial capacity for *Bartonella bacilliformis* and the agents of some arboviruses (SARAIVA et al, 2006).

Its transmission occurs through the bite of infected female phlebotomines, involving different species in close associations with parasites and reservoirs, making up the links in various transmission cycles that occur throughout the country. Since the 1980s, a process of geographical expansion of the transmission of the disease has been taking place, leading to its occurrence in all of the country's federal units today, with changes in the epidemiological profile of the disease (PENNA et al, 2011).

In Brazil, ATL has different epidemiological aspects, depending on the biogeographical characteristics of the regions where the disease is found. It can be found not only in forest regions, with abundant vegetation, favourable to the colonisation of infected psychodids and wild mammals, but also in deforested regions, with the adaptation of vectors and reservoirs to modified environments, in rural and urban areas, with peridomiciliary transmission. The presence of men and women with the same infection rate and patients in all age groups has also been recorded, and where no infected wild mammals have been found, domestic dogs seem to play an important role in extra-forest transmission (MAYWALD et al,1990).

The changes in the environment caused by the intense migration process, the growing urbanisation process and socio-economic pressures have led to the expansion of endemic areas and the appearance of new outbreaks. In this way, the phlebotomine species that somehow resist the adverse conditions are able to explore new environments, getting closer and closer to peridomiciles, facilitating the transmission of the disease (DIAS et *al,* 2007).

These latest findings suggest changes in the transmission pattern of the disease, probably due to changes in the habits of the mosquito vector, reinforcing the current importance of peridomiciliary or intradomiciliary transmission (PENNA et al, 2011).

In recent years, the significant increase in deforestation has favoured the adaptation of vectors to anthropogenic environments and, consequently, increased human exposure to the parasite. The circulation of *Leishmania* in domestic environments has favoured the emergence of a different profile for the transmission of the disease, which differs from the classic pattern and is associated with a wider range of activities (BARATA et al, 2011).

Leishmaniasis is on the increase due to serious changes in ecosystems, especially deforestation for population settlements, the opening of roads, irrigation projects, the construction of hydroelectric power stations and excessive urbanisation, among others. In addition, malnutrition, genetic susceptibility, acquired immunodeficiency syndrome and the parasite's resistance to pentavalent antimonials in several countries aggravate the situation (NUNES et *al,* 2006).

According to Tonelli and Freire (2000), ATL is primarily an enzootic disease of wild animals. Transmission to humans occurs when they enter areas where the disease occurs, making it zoonotic. There are currently two distinct epidemiological patterns in Brazil:

1) Epidemic outbreaks in areas of recent colonisation, associated with the clearing of forests to open roads or new population centres, etc., behaving as a zoonosis of wild animals and affecting people who interfere in the wild cycle. More common in the Amazon, they can also be seen in certain areas of the north-east.

1.1.1. hmaniasis in regions of old colonisation where there is no longer any deforestation. Dogs, horses and rodents seem to play an important role as reservoirs of the parasite. It is more common in the north-east and south-east.

2.5.4. Diagnosis and treatment

The first step in diagnosis should be to establish a history of exposure. It is important to distinguish the more innocuous cutaneous forms of leishmaniasis from the mucocutaneous forms, which are not usually self-limiting. Therapy for leishmaniasis is not benign and therefore the right diagnosis is crucial (WILSON & SANDE, 2004).

In the typical forms, the clinical diagnosis is made without difficulty, especially if the patient comes from endemic areas or has been in contact with forests in leishmaniasis zones. However, in general, this diagnosis requires confirmation or is established through laboratory tests (REY, 2002).

In 1926, Montenegro published a technique for isolating an antigen, which was named after him, from cultures of the parasite that had been inactivated by physical or chemical methods and showed a reliable intradermal reaction.

This reaction has been used extensively in epidemiological surveys and clinical diagnosis. It assesses the patient's delayed sensitivity, which is why it is used as a diagnostic technique. In epidemiological surveys or in monitoring vaccination programmes against ATL, it assesses infection even in the absence of disease. It consists of an intradermal injection of a suspension of Leishmania promastigotes at a concentration of 40 pg of nitrogen, a dose of 1.0 to 0.2 mL, on the anterior surface of the forearm, which will be read between 48 and 72 hours after the injection. The reading is considered positive when there is a papule at the injection site. The sensitivity of the test is around 85 to 97 per cent (TONELLI & FREIRE, 2000).

A positive response is obtained in 95% of proven cases of leishmaniasis. The test can be negative in recent cases (where finding the parasite under the microscope is usually easy), but in chronic cases it becomes the method of choice due to its high sensitivity and specificity (REY, 2002).

Histopathological examination is the fragment obtained from the skin by biopsy and submitted to routine histological techniques. The finding of amastigotes or a compatible inflammatory infiltrate can define or suggest the diagnosis (NEVES, 2001).

In Brazil and other New World countries, its importance lies not only in its high incidence and wide geographical distribution, but also in the possibility of it taking on forms that can cause destructive, disfiguring and also disabling lesions, with major repercussions in the individual's psychosocial field. Timely and appropriate treatment is of great importance to prevent the disease from progressing to more destructive and serious forms, such as the mucosal form (PENNA et al, 2011).

Broadly expanding geographically in Brazil, ATL is considered one of the most important dermatological infections, not only because of its frequency, but mainly because of the therapeutic difficulties, deformities and sequelae it can cause (DIAS et *al,* 2007).

The treatment of ATL was introduced by the Brazilian doctor Gaspar Vianna in 1912 with the use of the emetic antimonial Tartar. For many years, this drug was the only treatment in the world. Currently, a pentavalent antimonial is used, Glucantime - N-methyl glucamine antimoniate (NEVES, 2001).

The WHO (1990) recommends pentavalent antimonials as the first choice in the treatment of leishmaniasis, and the alternatives to the lack of response to these drugs are amphotericin B and pentamidine. Other drugs have been used, such as allopurinol, rifampicin, ketoconazole, itraconazole and mefloquine, but the results achieved were not consistent enough for them to be indicated. Amphotericin B is the drug of second choice, used when there is no response to treatment with pentavalent antimonials or when it is impossible to use them (TONELLI & FREIRE, 2000).

The drug should not be used in cardiac patients or pregnant women, as antimony can cause electrocardiographic changes and is also an abortifacient (NEVES, 2001).

There are also restrictions on the treatment of patients with heart disease, nephropathy, liver disease and Chagas disease, who need to be rigorously assessed and monitored in order to orientate their therapeutic behaviour (TONELLI & FREIRE, 2000).

ATL is considered a neglected disease. In general, it affects populations with low socioeconomic status, little political clout and little appeal for the pharmaceutical industry. The drugs currently used to treat this endemic disease often cause adverse effects. After clinical studies, the Ministry of Health approved the oral drug miltefosine for use in Brazil. In order to be implemented in the control programme, it is waiting for the laboratory that produces it to regularise its registration with ANVISA. This drug has been used in other countries that suffer from this endemic disease (PENNA et al, 2011).

2.5.5. Control and prevention of ATL

Controlling leishmaniasis is a priority for the World Health Organisation (WHO) and measures such as eliminating vectors with insecticides in the home, peridomicile and impregnated collars to prevent canine infection, as well as sacrificing infected dogs, have not had the expected impact (NUNES et *al,* 2006).

Municipalities are responsible for developing ATL control programmes, based on the standards and guidelines of the National Tegumentary Leishmaniasis Control Plan (PNCLT) in force. To this end, the need to adapt to existing local diversities is emphasised, especially in relation to Supervised Treatment (ST) (BRASIL, 2005).

The hierarchisation of services and their arrangement in networks is a process that is under construction in Brazil. Care networks are a set of units with different profiles and functions, organised in an articulated manner, responsible for the comprehensive provision of health services in a given region, understood as the territorial and population base that is self-sufficient up to the level of complexity that is defined, encompassing the geopolitical structure of the country or state, cities or a single city or part of it, reserving the specificities and peculiarities of each reality (JESUS & ASSIS, 2010).

In 2000, the Ministry of Health instituted the *Strategic Plan for the Implementation of the Tegumentary Leishmaniasis Control Plan in Brazil for the period 2001 to 2005,* which included partnerships with primary care services, mainly the Community Health Agents Programme (PACS) and the Family Health Programme (PSF), with the aim of expanding actions to control ATL in order to achieve greater detection and cure of cases of the disease (BRASIL, 2005).

In line with SUS guidelines, the process of decentralising care to basic health units (UBS) began in 2002 in the municipalities with the highest ATL detection rates, and was later extended to the others. Decentralisation aims to: facilitate the population's access to health services; encourage early diagnosis; improve patient follow-up by the Family Health Programme (PSF) teams; reduce the abandonment rate; identify risk factors; institute educational measures (LIMA *et al,* 2007).

As defined by the Organic Health Law (Law 8.080/90), epidemiological surveillance is "the set of activities that allows us to gather the indispensable information to know, at any time, the behaviour or natural history of diseases, as well as to detect or predict changes in their conditioning factors, with the aim of timely recommending the indicated and efficient measures that lead to the prevention and control of certain diseases" (PENNA et *al,* 2011, p. 01).

The American Tegumentary Leishmaniasis Surveillance Programme (PV-LTA) aims to diagnose and treat detected cases at an early stage in order to reduce the deformities caused by the disease.

The specific objectives of the PV-LTA are:

-identify and monitor territorial units of epidemiological relevance; investigate and characterise outbreaks; monitor severe forms with mucosal destruction; identify autochthonous cases early in areas considered non-endemic; reduce the number of cases in areas of household transmission; adopt relevant control measures, after epidemiological investigation, in areas of household transmission; monitor adverse events to medicines.

With the effective decentralisation of endemic diseases (cholera, dengue, tuberculosis, meningitis, trachoma, leishmaniasis, among others), the State and Municipal Health Departments must take on the role of controlling the diseases prevalent in their respective regions, as well as coordinating, programming and planning care for leishmaniasis sufferers (BRASIL, 2000).

It is in this context that compulsorily notifiable dermatological diseases such as leishmaniasis are monitored, with a view to formulating and evaluating health policies, plans and programmes, supporting the decision-making process and contributing to improving the population's health situation.

Today, diseases and outbreaks follow the rules of the new International Health Regulations (IHR), approved by the World Assembly of Health Ministers in 2005 and ratified by Legislative Decree No. 395 of June 2009 of the Brazilian Federal Senate. To keep in line with the IHR, Ministerial Ordinance No. 2472 of 31 August 2010, containing 44 events, standardises compulsory notification in our country for a large list of diseases and illnesses (PENNA et *al,* 2011).

Actions to control ATL should be the subject of a continuous programme aimed at: diagnosing the patient, by meeting demand and actively searching for cases, providing supplies for complementary diagnosis, investigating outbreaks and properly recording their occurrence; standardised therapeutic guidance, providing medication and monitoring the patient, and epidemiological investigation of outbreaks and adoption of the relevant prophylactic measures.

In order to define the strategies and the need for control actions for each area of ATL to be worked on, the epidemiological aspects and their determinants must be taken into account. This requires: a description of ATL cases according to age, sex, clinical form, place of transmission (household or extra-household); the spatial distribution of cases; investigation in the area of transmission to find out and try to establish determinants, such as: the presence of animals, in order to verify possible food sources and favourable ecotopes for the establishment of the vector; the presence of rubbish, which could attract synanthropic animals to the vicinity of the household; housing conditions, which facilitate access for the vector; delimitation and characterisation of the area of transmission.

This research will indicate the need to adopt measures to control ATL, highlighting that early diagnosis and appropriate treatment of human cases, as well as educational activities, should be prioritised in all situations.

Patients can be cared for through spontaneous demand at health units, active search for cases in areas of transmission, when indicated by epidemiological surveillance or the family health team, or in risk areas where it is difficult for the population to access health units.

In order to structure and organise diagnostic and treatment services, as well as to guarantee the quality of care for patients with ATL, it is necessary to: identify the health units and the professionals who will be assisting the patients. It is recommended that at least one doctor, one nurse and one nursing assistant be appointed to each team; define the laboratory and the professional from the same or a reference health unit who will carry out at least the IDRM reading and the parasitological examination; train the professionals who will make up the multi-professional team at the basic health units and laboratories or referral centres in laboratory and clinical diagnosis and treatment; sensitise the network's professionals to clinical suspicion, involving all the family health teams; supply the health units with the materials and supplies needed for diagnosis and treatment; establish patient care routines, offering the necessary conditions for monitoring patients, with a view to reducing abandonment and complications caused mainly by adverse effects of medication; establish the flow of referrals and counter-referrals for clinical and laboratory diagnosis and treatment; implement or improve the flow of information of interest to surveillance and assistance; regularly evaluate and publicise the actions carried out by the services, as well as the epidemiological situation of ATL; investigate all patients with ATL who have died, filling in the appropriate investigation form in order to identify the probable causes of death (BRASIL, 2000).

To date, there are no definitively effective control measures to combat ATL. Vaccines are being developed in several countries, including Brazil, but they still require further studies before they can be released for use by the population. A vaccine developed by Mayrink, at the Federal University of Minas Gerais - UFMG, with protection of around 60%, has been commercialised and exported by the company Biobrás to different countries (TONELLI & FREIRE, 2000).

In 1961, Professor Wilson Mayrink began studies on the prophylaxis of Visceral Leishmaniasis in Caratinga (MG). Since 1961, his efforts have resulted in the control of kala-azar, and in the 1980s he began coordinating a major study to test the efficacy of the vaccine against ATL.

According to Mayrink, "Leishmaniasis only continues to grow to this day and it can only be prevented with a vaccine. However

American Tegumentary Leishmaniasis practically only affects the poorest population, and because of this, there is little investment in field research and less attention from funding bodies in this field".

The researcher's project is continuing with positive results for the population. The vaccine is produced by him in the Parasitology department at UFMG, tested and approved by the Pharmacy school and CETEC. Despite the good results obtained over the years, the vaccine is only approved by the Ministry of Health for therapeutic use and not for preventing the disease (Available at: http:// revista.fapemig.br).

However, although there is no vaccination programme as a preventative mechanism, there are some measures that can be taken to avoid the risks of transmission.

Collective measures should also be encouraged, such as: pruning trees to increase sunlight, in order to reduce shading of the ground and avoid favourable conditions (temperature and humidity) for the development of phlebotomine larvae; in potential areas of transmission, a buffer zone of 400 to 500 metres between homes and the forest is suggested.

Individual preventive measures should also be taken: use of repellents when exposed to environments where the vectors can usually be found; avoid exposure at times when the vector is active (dusk and night); use of fine mesh mosquito nets (mesh size 1.2 to 1. 5 and denier 40 to 100); environmental management by cleaning up backyards and land in order to change the environmental conditions that favour the establishment of breeding sites.5 mesh size and denier 40 to 100), as well as shading doors and windows; environmental management by cleaning up backyards and plots of land in order to change the environmental conditions that favour the establishment of breeding sites for immature forms of the vector; proper disposal of organic waste in order to prevent the approach of commensal mammals such as marsupials and rodents, probable sources of infection for phlebotomines; periodic cleaning of domestic animal shelters; keeping domestic animals away from the home at night in order to reduce the attraction of phlebotomines to this environment (BRASIL, 2000).

Health education activities must be included in all the services that carry out ATL surveillance and control actions, requiring the effective involvement of multi-professional and multi-institutional teams with a view to working together in the different service provision units (BRASIL, 2005).

These activities should include disseminating information to the population about the occurrence of ATL in the region, municipality or locality, advising them to recognise clinical signs and seek out services for diagnosis and treatment when there is a suspected case; training teams from community health agent programmes (Pacs), family health (PSF), environmental and epidemiological surveillance and other professionals from related areas for early diagnosis and appropriate treatment; establishing inter-institutional partnerships to implement health-related actions, especially public cleaning and the proper disposal of organic waste; implementing a health education programme, developing information, education and communication activities at local, regional and municipal level (BRASIL, 2000). I think they prioritise diagnosis and treatment first, when it should be prevention!

In addition to the above-mentioned measures, the Epidemiological Surveillance Guide also presents new tools: team training, encompassing technical knowledge, psychological aspects and professional practice in relation to the disease and the sick; adoption of preventive measures, considering knowledge of the disease, attitudes and practices of the population (clientele), related to people's living and working conditions; establishment of a dynamic relationship between the professional's knowledge and the experience of the different social strata, through a global understanding of the health/disease process, in which social, economic, political and cultural factors intervene (BRASIL, 2005).

2.5.6. The role of municipalities and epidemiological surveillance

Until 1986, patients with ATL were cared for by health agents from the now defunct Superintendence of Public Health Campaigns (SUCAM). When the agents in charge of malaria surveillance travelled around the municipalities, they learnt about the cases and gave the medication to people suspected of being infected with Leishmania. Thus, treatment was carried out at random, without laboratory diagnosis and medical follow-up (LIMA et al, 2007).

In line with SUS guidelines, the process of decentralising care to basic health units (UBS) began in 2002 in the municipalities with the highest ATL detection rates, and was later extended to the others. Decentralisation aims to: facilitate the population's access to health services; encourage early diagnosis; improve patient follow-up by the PSF teams; reduce the abandonment rate; identify risk factors; institute educational measures (BRASIL, 2005).

In 2002, patients were decentralised to the municipalities where they lived, with the aim of facilitating access to diagnosis and treatment. The process began gradually, initially including the municipalities with the highest prevalence of the disease.

In 2003, decentralisation reached all the municipalities and care began to be provided in the UBS. Several stages of training were carried out for the municipal service teams, including practical monitoring at the reference outpatient clinic (LIMA et *al,* 2007).

The current challenges for ATL are: a) expanding the health network for early diagnosis and adequate treatment of cases; b) implementing surveillance actions in territorial units; c) expanding entomological surveillance actions; d) increasing investments in the search for drugs with better efficacy, safety, low cost, ease of administration and sustainability; e) maintaining surveillance of the adverse effects of drugs; f) investigating and assessing deaths (PENNA et al, 2011).

It is also a serious problem from an economic point of view, as the cost of implementing leishmaniasis control is high and often unsuccessful. One of the main factors contributing to this inefficiency is related to the fact that the leishmaniasis control programmes operated by the various local health systems were conceived within the same conceptual frameworks and strict logic that characterise endemic disease control programmes in Brazil. These are not effective, partly because they do not recognise or fail to incorporate into the approach to the health-disease process the network of social representations engendered in the daily lives of the affected populations (SILVA, 2007).

The epidemiological surveillance sector aims to diagnose and treat detected cases. The role of surveillance in controlling ATL is discussed below.

ATL is a compulsorily notifiable disease in which every confirmed case must be notified and investigated by the health services using the investigation form standardised by the Notifiable Diseases Information System (SINAN). Its registration is important for knowledge, investigation, epidemiological classification (autochthonous or imported case) and follow-up (BRASIL, 2006).

The data collection instrument is the SINAN epidemiological form, which contains the essential elements to be collected in a routine investigation. All the fields on this form must be carefully filled in, even when the information is negative or ignored. Other items and observations should be included, according to the needs and peculiarities of each situation (BRASIL, 2005).

Detection of ATL cases can occur through spontaneous demand at health units; active search for cases in transmission areas; home visits by professionals from the Community Health Agents Programme (PACS) and PSF; referrals of suspects by the basic health network.

Once a case of ATL has been detected, epidemiological investigation is generally necessary in order to: know the epidemiological characteristics of the case (clinical form, age and sex) and economic activity related to transmission; identify whether the patient comes from an endemic area or is a new focus of transmission; carry out an active search for new cases and characterise them clinically and laboratory; carry out entomological research, if necessary, to define the species of sandflies involved in transmission; assess the probable site of infection (LPI), to verify the need to adopt chemical control measures (BRASIL, 2000).

It is in this context that the present study on ATL control policies in the municipality of Montes Claros was carried out.

CHAPTER 3

METHODOLOGY

This chapter consists of eight sections. In the first we will characterise the research, in the second we will present the type of research, in the third we will look at the field of research, in the fourth we will describe our sample/population, in the fifth we will present the instrument used for data collection, in the sixth section we will describe the procedure used for data collection, in the seventh we will detail the treatment of the data and finally, in the eighth section, we will reflect on the ethical aspects.

3.1. Research characterisation

Three procedures were used: bibliographical, documentary and field sources. The bibliographic source is the survey of the subject concerning the research in literature.

Traditional bibliographical research was carried out by searching the literature for articles related to the subject, on academic sites such as SCIELO, MEDLINE, LILACS and BVS. The main keywords used in this search were: "Public Policies, Public Health Policies, Economy and Health, American Tegumentary Leishmaniasis and Control of American Tegumentary Leishmaniasis".

This is a qualitative evaluation study. Although there are still debates about the appropriateness of using quantitative and qualitative methods in judging health services, the qualitative approach is recognised by several authors as being of great relevance for understanding the analogies between the degree of implementation and the political and organisational situation (GONTIJO et *al,* 2012).

The qualitative approach was chosen due to the complexity of the health field and the nature of the object of study, since, as Minayo (2007) points out, this type of research allows us to ascertain the meanings attributed by the subjects to the fact of their practices, as well as aiming to delve deeper into the world of meanings, human relationships, attitudes, beliefs and values. According to the author, this approach is not concerned with quantification, but rather with understanding and explaining the dynamics of the phenomenon *(apud* CAMOSSA et al., 2012).

A qualitative approach was used, since this study was not concerned with enumerating and/or measuring the events studied, but with capturing the reality of the phenomenon.

As a rule of qualitative methodology, it is essential that the researcher does not influence the participant's answers, so that they feel free to express their line of thought and are able to externalise the mental classes they use (GASPAROTTO et *al* 2012).

Qualitative research is an attempt to understand the meanings and characteristics of a situation, rather than producing quantitative measures of characteristics or behaviours (BONACIM & ARAÚJO, 2011).

The qualitative research methodology takes into account the perception of individuals and is built on the product of the discourses/verbalisations of social interpreters directly involved with the subject. The qualitative approach to thinking about the issues being studied allows us to take hold of the interviewees' individual perceptions and modify them into a more coherent and consistent discourse, thus being able to obtain the social aspects indicative of the themes being worked on in this group of individuals (CASTRO et al, 2010).

According to Gonçalvez Rey (2002, p.51), the positions taken by qualitative research allow the search for "knowledge of a complex object: subjectivity, whose elements are simultaneously involved in different processes that make up the whole, which change depending on the context in which the concrete subject is expressed".

Tasks with intricate questions do not give the researcher an exact, *a priori* sense of the paths the research will follow. Flexibility in the research direction process is one of the characteristics of qualitative research (ANDRADE, 2007).

González Rey (2005, p.18) emphasises: "to take the new as a new form of pre-existing knowledge is to castrate what is new about it". Thus, the trajectory of the research depends on the context in which it takes place, without losing sight of the fact that the researcher influences the research situation and is also influenced by it.

Qualitative methods are procedures in the human sciences that study, specify and evaluate phenomena (visible or hidden). These phenomena are essentially not capable of being measured (a belief, a representation, a personal style of relating to others, a strategy in the face of a problem, a decision-making procedure...), they have the unique characteristics of "human facts".

The "quality" of phenomena does not appear immediately to experience, nor is it constructed through induction. The qualitative approach therefore sets out to clarify and recognise the difficult expressions of the constitution of subjectivity, unlike the "quantitative" intention of prediction, description and control (HOLANDA, 2006).

Gonçalvez Rey (2002) adds that, given the active participation of the researcher - a characteristic of qualitative research - their narration and cultural situation should be understood as elements of great significance in the research, as they mark a singularity that is the expression of the heritage and plasticity of the subjective phenomenon.

Another important characteristic of qualitative research is emphasised by Martins and Bicudo (2005). According to the authors, qualitative research seeks a reserved understanding of what it studies, since the focus of its attention is orientated towards the particular, the singular, aiming to understand the phenomena studied, which only appear when situated.

The research seeks to maintain a stable relationship between four basic guidelines: theory, the empirical moment, the instruments and the process of constructing and explaining information with the production of knowledge, in a continuous development established by both the researcher and the researched. Thus, qualitative research does not only fulfil an instrumental sense, it is epistemological and theoretical and supports unique processes of knowledge construction (ANDRADE, 2007).

González Rey (2002) observes that researchers who simply focus on methodological differences generally differentiate between qualitative and quantitative research only at the level of techniques.

For Amatuzzi (2003) and Holanda (2006), when looking for unique information, the researcher removes the focus from theory, harbouring the empirical as access to knowledge production and the possibility of building new theories, especially since theory is a living process, in development and construction.

According to Gonçalvez Rey (2002, p.51), the spaces occupied by qualitative research allow for the investigation of "knowledge of a complex object: subjectivity, whose elements are implicated simultaneously in different constitutive processes of the whole, which change in the face of the context in which the concrete subject is expressed".

It is considered that the subjectivity in the experience of the subjects involved with ATL is both included in the process and will imply the expected results, and should always be included in the analysis. The ideas and attitudes of the health professionals, as well as those of the participating managers, are part of the representations about the control of ATL and have implications for the proposal of this work.

3.2. Type of research

In the different types of qualitative research (such as the ethnographic model, heuristic research, hermeneutics, grounded-theory, historiographical research, case studies, biographical research and phenomenological research), the researcher and the subject are thinkers. The specificity of qualitative research refers to the investigation of aspects of the subject's reality, taking into account that these aspects are apprehended by research subjects (ANDRADE, 2007).

Creswell (1998) points in the direction of five "traditions" in qualitative research: biography (or biographical study), phenomenological study, "grounded theory", ethnography and case study (apud HOLANDA, 2006).

We can start from this definition by Creswell to characterise the qualitative method in research and point out the phenomenological modality that was applied to this research.

We used the phenomenological method, which according to Holanda (2006), is a methodology that presents qualitative methods as differentiated models of empirical approach, specifically aimed at so-called "human phenomena", in other words, as methods that escape the classic connection with empirical aspects such as measurement and control.

The phenomenological method, which Creswell (1998) considers to be *the* "description of the lived experiences" of various subjects about a concept or phenomenon, with the aim of seeking out the "essential" structure or the "invariant" elements of the phenomenon, in other words, its "central meaning" (HOLANDA, 2006).

Phenomenological research therefore involves a return to experience in order to obtain comprehensive descriptions that will provide support for analysing the phenomenon being researched.

Amatuzzi (1996, p.5), quoted by Andrade (2007), states that phenomenological research is a form of qualitative research that "designates the study of the lived, or of immediate pre-reflective experience, with the aim of describing its meaning; or any study that takes the lived as a clue or method.

In short, it's research that deals with the meaning of the experience."

Creswell (1998) points out that the character of the phenomenological method can be challenging. As well as the researcher needing a solid grounding in the philosophical principles of phenomenology, the collaborators in the study need to be carefully chosen because they are individuals who experience the phenomenon. Another challenge is for the researcher to hold personal experiences, a goal that is always present and never achieved to perfection. A fourth challenge is deciding how their personal experiences are placed in the study (apud ANDRADE, 2007).

But what is phenomenology anyway? The term Phenomenology comes from the Greek words phainomenon (that which shows itself) and logos (science or study). In this etymological sense, Phenomenology is the study or science of phenomena. Phenomenon, in its most generic sense, means everything that appears, manifests or reveals itself, which is why the field of Phenomenology is extensive and practically unlimited (MORA, 2001; ABBAGNANO, 2003; JAPIASSU & MARCONDES, 2006).

Phenomenology is the science that applies itself to the study of phenomena: objects, events and happenings in reality. Phenomenology presents "a truth, in parts and in moments, and never in its total transparency, because it is doubt, not certainty, that motivates us to the incessant search for truth". It is necessary to remember that "truth is a movement in constitution, not a state" (MOREIRA, 2004, p. 449).

Reduction is the common resource used by Phenomenology to reach the essence of the phenomenon, making it understandable and validating it scientifically. The first step for this to happen is to change from the natural attitude - which Husserl (1992) called common sense - to the phenomenological attitude. As Forghieri (1993, p.15) explains, this change in attitude makes it possible to visualise the subject's world as a phenomenon, "or as constituting a totality, within which the world and the subject reveal themselves reciprocally as meanings" (apud ANDRADE, 2007).

From this perspective, the phenomenological researcher, according to Moreira (2004), when practising reduction, must interrupt their own thoughts and interests, and thus be open to any type of content or subject that may arise in their research. As a result, it is common for phenomenological research to achieve new, totally unforeseen results. In the author's opinion, this is research that is open to new and creative possibilities for understanding the object of study.

The phenomenological method, according to Creswell (1998), is the description of the lived experiences of the research subjects about a concept or phenomenon, with the aim of seeking out the essential structure of the phenomenon, i.e. its central meaning (apud ANDRADE, 2007).

In short, the phenomenological method, according to Holanda (2003), should seek to access the essence, the eidos of the phenomenon studied, which can be achieved by using a method that considers the three basic elements of phenomenology. The first element is phenomenological reduction, which is the suspension of the researcher's judgements in relation to the subject being researched, enabling them to access the subject's truth. The second element is intersubjectivity, which is the relationship established between the subject-researcher and the subject-researched - two people with their own histories who meet in order to understand a phenomenon. The third element mentioned by the author is the return to the lived experience, in which the research subject returns to their lived world, their history, through their interview.

For all of these reasons, we opted for the phenomenological method, since our central objective is the meaning of the research subjects' knowledge of the essential element of LTA control, with the aim of achieving the fundamental composition of this phenomenon, that is, its main constitution, by understanding the research subjects' experience of this public policy episode.

3.3. Field of research

In the specific case of this research, data was collected using the Epidemiological Surveillance sector, Basic Health Units (UBS's), public hospitals and, finally, the Zoonoses sector of the municipality of Montes Claros - MG as the field of investigation.

We therefore consider it pertinent to characterise the Municipality of Montes Claros, since it is part of the field of research. We will then describe the role played by each of the fields of research.

The municipality of Montes Claros is located in the northern region of the state of Minas Gerais. It is located in the Upper Middle São Francisco basin, in the "Drought Polygon" area. The municipality covers an area of approximately 4,135 km^2 . It is located at an altitude of 638 metres and its position is determined by the following geographical coordinates: 16°42'16" south latitude and 43°49'13" west longitude, 420 km from the capital of Minas Gerais. The climate is tropical semi-humid, with an average temperature of around 25°C and a long dry season (approximately five months a year). Climatological data indicates annual rainfall of around 520 mm, with rainfall occurring between October and March, and relative humidity ranging from 52 to 80%.

Epidemiological surveillance is the sector responsible for action on disease transmission, educational and administrative measures and vaccination. It covers everything from case detection, confirmation, recording of treatment, recording of basic variables, flow of care and information, cure, abandonment and regular treatment (BASANO & CAMARGO, 2004).

As defined in the Organic Health Law (Law 8.080/90), epidemiological surveillance is the set of activities that allows us to gather the information needed to know, at any time, the behaviour or natural history of diseases, as well as to detect or predict changes in their conditioning factors, with the aim of providing timely advice, on a firm basis, on the appropriate and efficient measures to prevent and control certain diseases (BRASIL, 2007).

The UBS's are part of the family health strategy or family health plan, better known as the Family Health Centre. Its model is the reorientation of care, operationalised through the deployment of multi-professional teams in basic health units. These teams are responsible for monitoring a defined number of families, located in a geographical area adjacent to the unit. The teams work on health promotion, prevention, recovery and rehabilitation of the most common diseases and illnesses; they are also responsible for accompanying families during and after treatment (OLIVEIRA, 2011).

Public hospitals are health establishments with differentiated services, which have inpatient, outpatient (consultation and emergency) and diagnostic and therapeutic facilities, with the aim of providing the population with curative and rehabilitative medical care, while also being responsible for collaborating in disease prevention, teaching and scientific research (SAÚDE, 2001).

The aim of university hospitals is also to provide health services. In addition to providing medical care, they also provide teaching and research activities and should be a benchmark in cutting-edge technology (BONACIM & ARAÚJO, 2011).

Zoonosis Control Centres (CCZs) are public health units whose fundamental aim is to prevent and control zoonoses (such as rabies, dengue fever, Chagas disease and leishmaniasis) by developing health and epidemiological surveillance systems. They fulfil their roles by controlling populations of domestic animals (dogs, cats and large animals) and controlling populations of synanthropic animals (bats, pigeons, rats, mosquitoes, bees, among others). This task is based on educational work, seeking to enlighten and count on the collaboration and participation of society as a whole, complemented by legal and fiscal actions. Zoonosis Control Centres are also allowed to euthanise animals, as long as they use humane methods (available at http://www.saude.rio.rj .gov.br/).

3.4. Population/Sample

Field research should be given a great deal of attention, as the criteria for choosing the sample (the people who will be chosen as examples of a certain situation), the way in which the data will be collected and the criteria for analysing the data obtained should be pointed out.

The production of narratives must define certain procedures, such as who, when and how many subjects will be interviewed. It should also be remembered that the method discussed here produces a large volume of collected material (GIL, 2005).

According to Minayo (2006, p. 197) "one of the criteria that must be taken into account in the process of defining the qualitative sample is: to clearly define the social group on which the central question of the research falls and to centre the focus of the interviews on them". In our case, we will be studying a social group, which are employees working in health service units, involved in the prevention, diagnosis, treatment and control of ATL, located in the municipality of Montes Claros, on whom we will focus our interviews.

The universe of the research was then selected: health professionals (doctors, nurses and nursing technicians) who work in the UBSs and public hospitals of

Montes Claros. The UBS's were selected according to location, covering various neighbourhoods, according to the management distributed in the municipality, totalling 7 health units. This broad spectrum of selected units was intended to guarantee sample heterogeneity. Public hospitals were also selected, totalling 4 hospitals: the University Hospital (2), the Aroldo Tourinho Hospital (1) and the Alfeu de Quadros Hospital (1). The population also included professionals working in the Epidemiological Surveillance sector of the Montes Claros Municipal Health Department and the Zoonosis Control Centre sector, which is responsible for controlling ATL in the municipality. The total population of health professionals in the municipality of Montes Claros is around 8,500 individuals.

The inclusion criteria for taking part in the research were as follows:

- exercise professional activity in the health area;

-be involved in any of the processes of prevention, diagnosis, treatment and control of ATL;

-agree to take part in the research by signing an informed consent form.

The sample of health professionals included doctors, nurses and nursing technicians who attended to patients during their working hours in the selected units. The aim was to have professionals who were representative of the different units and to have a set of key informants in the context of our investigation. This sample therefore consisted of a convenience sample. The surveillance professionals included those responsible for attending to patients and referring them to the network services offered by the Municipal Health Department of São Paulo.

Montes Claros, including the notification of ATL cases and, in the Zoonosis Control Centre sector, the health agent was included because he has an active and direct role in the control of leishmaniasis in the municipality of Montes Claros.

In this way, this population was the most suitable for providing exploratory and preliminary data, so that we could identify important issues in this research that would help to achieve our proposed objectives.

The sample involving the UBS's and Hospitals was made up of 11 health professionals, 7 from the Health Units, made up of 4 nurses, 2 nursing technicians and 1 doctor, and 4 from the hospitals, made up of 3 nurses and 1 nursing technician. The sample in the surveillance sector was made up of the Director of Health Surveillance, the Coordinator of Epidemiological Surveillance and a professional Nursing Technician, making up 3 employees. And finally, at the Zoonosis Control Centre, the sample was made up of 1 health worker. The total sample thus consisted of 15 professionals, around 0.125% of the population.

The exclusion criterion was not agreeing to take part in the research at the time of data collection. Excluded from the epidemiology sector were professionals who usually worked with the task of notifying diseases (information system), working exclusively with SINAN, which is the investigation form standardised by the Sistema de Informação de Agravos de Notificacão (Notifiable Diseases Information System). The purpose of this system would be epidemiological classification (autochthonous or imported case) and case follow-up, so these employees would not be able to express themselves in relation to ATL, in terms of the elements of significance of this research.

3.5. Data collection instrument

One of the resources widely used to gain an understanding of the phenomenon or reality being studied is the interview. In the interview, the researcher can explore the lived experience and the meaning that the lived world has for the interviewee or interviewees, and understand how different people experience a certain condition that is common to them. There are various interview models and this paper will discuss the interview using the phenomenological method that was used to interpret the text.

For our research, we used semi-structured interviews with a script of questions.

This type of interview "is developed from a fixed list of questions, the order and wording of which remains the same for all interviewees", according to Gil (2007, p.123).

Our interview consisted of 8 questions, organised into 2 parts. The first part includes socio-demographic characterisation questions; the second part includes questions covering all aspects of ATL control in Montes Claros and the human and financial resources involved (Appendix 1 - Interview script).

The semi-structured interview was chosen because "this type of interview is linked to the expectation that the views of the interviewees are more likely to be expressed in an interview situation with a relatively open plan than in a standardised interview, as Flick (2004, p.89) points out.

An important characteristic of the semi-structured interview as a data collection technique in qualitative research is the character of interaction that permeates it, i.e. the relationship that is created provides an environment of reciprocal influence between the questioner and the answerer, with no rigid order of questions to be followed by the researcher. The interviewee discusses the proposed topic according to the information they have and also based on their impressions and social values (SOUZA, 2008).

For Amatuzzi (2003), the subjects are called collaborators, because the author understands that phenomenological research does not deal with subjects who provide information, but collaborators who, together, approach the subject. It is based on the methodological hypothesis that the collaborator is the one who knows best about their experience, while the researcher sets out to learn from those who have already lived or are living the experience about which they want to improve their knowledge. Both are transformed by this exchange.

3.5.1. Pre-test

A pre-test of the interview was carried out with 2 epidemiological surveillance officials in March 2012. The interviews took place without incident, and the respondents understood the questions asked. There was no need to rephrase the questions, so the provisional version became the definitive version, with an application time of 36'14 minutes.

In this investigation, the categories analysed were: verification of the respondents' knowledge of disease control policies; strategies used in this control, resources used, implementation of decentralisation, treatment resources, effectiveness of the measures; the opinion of the sector's employees on the care provided by health professionals and the supply of health units relating to ATL; the employees' perception of the evolution of the disease and investigation into the municipality's human and financial resources involved in ATL control.

3.6. Data collection procedure

All the research procedures followed the ethical principles contained in the National Health Council's Guidelines and Regulatory Norms for Research Involving Human Beings, Resolution No. 196/96.

From the point of view of individuals and communities, this Resolution incorporates the four basic references of bioethics: autonomy, non-maleficence, beneficence and justice, among others, and aims to ensure the rights and duties that concern the scientific community, research subjects and the State.

The ethicality of research involving human beings implies: a) the free and informed consent of the target individuals and the protection of vulnerable groups and the legally incapable. In this sense, research involving human beings should always treat them with dignity, respect their autonomy and defend their vulnerability; b) weigh up risks and benefits, both actual and potential, individual and collective, committing to maximum benefits and minimum harm and risk; c) guarantee that foreseeable damage will be avoided; d) social relevance of the research with significant advantages for the research subjects and minimisation of the burden for vulnerable subjects, which guarantees equal consideration of the interests involved, without losing the sense of its socio-humanitarian purpose (justice and equity) (Available at http://www.bioetica.ufrgs.br/res19696.htm).

The consent form was drawn up with the aim of clarifying the purpose of the study and preserving the anonymity of the interviewees. Consent to participate was obtained by reading, clarifying and signing the informed consent form.

In order to guarantee the anonymity of the research subjects, the interviews were numbered according to the sequence in which they took place.

The data collection phase took place between September and October 2012. The place and date for the interviews were scheduled with the employees by mobile phone, and they were informed about the subject of the interview and its objectives.

After scheduling the interviews, we went to the workplace of each of the interviewees and carried out the interviews, which were recorded in full, since the discourse is important for exploring the phenomenon.

The 15 interviews took place in the service environment, at the interviewees' place of work, in order to more clearly understand the context of their information. The interviews lasted between 14'20 and 32'54 minutes.

The commitment of both parties, according to González Rey (2005), is fundamental to achieving the research objective. However, some problems can arise: the fear of the person coming into contact with wounds that are still open, the fear of talking about intimacies, the confrontation of their values, lack of trust in the researcher, lack of interest in the research, among others. Any impasse in the interview needs to be explained so that the process of knowledge can continue. Otherwise, there is a risk of losing the commitment and complicity of the pair. In our study, the interviews went smoothly and there were no embarrassing situations.

3.7. Data processing

Once the interview had been recorded, the first step was to transcribe the material, which is the transition from the oral form to written language, in a way that is faithful to what was contained in the recording. In total, the 15 interviews produced around 3h50' of recorded material. The information was organised using Microsoft WORD 2010.

The data collected was submitted to content analysis in order to achieve a deeper understanding of the phenomenon, beyond the descriptive scope of the content.

It was considered that everything in a narrative has meaning. In it, the subject offers events, explains them, expounds, restates ideas and contradicts himself, structuring his reflection throughout the speech. For this reason, however complete an analysis of the vertical whole of the discourse may be, in order for it to be effective, it is necessary to carry it out horizontally, since the meaning is not at the end of the narrative, it runs through it.

Gontijo et *al* (2012) also set out the stages that corresponded to our interview. The first stage involved analysing each interview separately. In this stage, the first moment is vertical reading, looking for the overall meaning of each interview and getting to know the "tone" of the interview. At this point, the researcher summarises the subjects covered, as a first approximation of the content. In the second stage, called "horizontal reading", the text of each interview was divided into sequences numbered in ascending order, in a process of textual "deconstruction", revealing the statements that point to the field of definitions for the person speaking about each object of discourse.

In the second stage, the "reconstruction" of the interview was carried out, when the subject's objects, explanations and points of view were regrouped, analysing the same subject addressed in the entire report, in order to locate, monitor and report on the categorisation work carried out by the interviewee himself. Reconstruction around the objects is indispensable because they are scattered throughout the speech, and the discursive process always involves going back and forth to present and justify them.

The third stage of the work involved, firstly, finding what was common and what was discordant in the categories explained by the group of interviewees, deepening the classification of the meanings explained about the objects in focus, in a so-called transversal reading. The second step was theorisation, in which the categories that emerged from the analysis of the interviews were deepened by the researcher's readings and theoretical reflections, allowing for comparison with other findings and theories from other researchers (GONTIJO et al, 2012).

Gomes (1997, p.328) clearly summarises the stages of data processing using the phenomenological method: "Initially, we have the raw data consisting of the interview protocols. At this point, this set of protocols functions as a crude description. The task of questioning these protocols and organising this material into comprehensive units is then reduction. The writing of a final text (...) *is* interpretation" *(apud* ANDRADE, 2007).

After systematically analysing the results, they were transformed into information on the Control of American Tegumentary Leishmaniasis in the Municipality of Montes Claros - MG.

The following categories emerged from the analysis process: knowledge about ATL and the priority given to the disease in the municipality; incidence and diagnosis of the disease; development of actions to control the disease; strategies related to the disease; decentralisation of services and resources earmarked for

ATL control.

CHAPTER 4

RESULTS AND DISCUSSION

The presentation and discussion of the results is organised into two sub-chapters: the first will characterise the sample and the second will describe the categories that emerged in the interviews, which had ATL control policies as their underlying theme, followed by a discussion comparing or confirming the findings with similar subjects and/or using studies carried out in Brazil or in countries with similar characteristics.

The sub-chapter dealing with ATL control policies is organised according to the subcategories of analysis: Interviewees' knowledge of ATL and priority given to the disease, the incidence of the disease in Montes Claros, diagnosis of the disease, control actions and their effectiveness, degree of participation in discussing and defining ATL control actions, evaluation of control actions by basic health units (BHUs), involvement of health workers in ATL control, strategies used in ATL control, decentralisation of services, human and material resources and monetary resources allocated to ATL control.

4.1. Characterisation of the sample

The sample will be characterised in terms of gender, age, education, profession, professional category and length of professional career (Table 2).

There was a predominance of women among the interviewees (11), and their ages ranged from 22 to 52. The interviewees' level of education ranged from high school to master's degree, with the majority (10) having higher education. As for the profession of the interviewees, the majority are nurses, followed by nursing technicians, with only one doctor and one biologist. Most of the professionals hold positions in line with their professions, except for one nurse who is the director of Health Surveillance and one biologist who is the coordinator of Epidemiological Surveillance. Career length ranged from 11 months to 15 years, with the majority having between 3 and 6 years of professional experience.

Table 2 - Characterisation of the sample of interviewees

Interviewee	Sex	Age	Education	Profession	Category in profession	Time in career
1	F	30	Superior	Nursing	UBS nurse*	4 years
2	F	30	High school	Nursing technician	UBS Nursing Technician	6 years
3	M	52	High school	Community agent	Zoonoses Health Agent	15 years
4	F	28	High school	Nursing technician	Hospital Nursing Technician	2 years
5	F	36	High school	Nursing technician	UBS Nursing Technician	3 years
6	F	25	Superior	Nursing	Hospital Nurse	11 months
7	F	22	Superior	Nursing	UBS nurse	4 months
8	F	32	High school	Nursing technician	Nursing technician in the EV sector**	3 years
9	F	51	Superior	Nursing	Director of health surveillance	12 years old
10	M	35	Superior	Bachelor of Biology	VE Coordinator	3 years
11	F	27	Superior	Nursing	UBS nurse	3 years
12	F	25	Superior	Medicine	UBS doctor	8 months
13	M	28	Postgraduate studies	Nursing	UBS nurse	5 years
14	F	36	Superior	Nursing	Hospital Nurse	12 years old
15	M	28	Superior	Nursing	Hospital Nurse	7 years

Source: According to the interview
*UBS: Basic Health Unit **VE: Epidemiological Surveillance

4.2. LTA control policies

In this subchapter we will describe and analyse the emerging subcategories resulting from the content analysis, in the order already indicated.

4.2.1 - Interviewees' knowledge of ATL and priority given to the disease

We began by asking the interviewees if they had ever heard of ATL, and all the interviewees said they were familiar with the disease. As for their opinion on the priority given to ATL within the municipality's health framework, **the vast majority of** interviewees (12) believe that ATL is prioritised **(yes)** in the municipality of Montes Claros, the most suggestive example of which is the quote from interviewee E8:

"Yes, because it's a disease that can affect an entire population if there's no vigilance."

Only three interviewees believe that ATL is **not** prioritised, justifying this tendency by the existence of more serious diseases that require more attention. This is the case with interviewee E10, whose quote follows:

"Not as a priority, because there are other diseases of greater interest. ATL wouldn't be the main disease in the municipality, there are other diseases that *need more care, more priorities."* (E10)

According to some authors, the three low-priority responses can be explained by negligence in combating the disease. According to Hotez et *al* (2008), several of the world's most important Neglected Tropical Diseases (NTDs) occur in Brazil. However, the burden of these diseases differs by region. The number of humans affected by NTDs is higher in areas of greater poverty. There is a direct relationship between the prevalence of these diseases and the human development index (HDI). There is a high prevalence of NTDs in Brazil and most of them occur in poor regions, mainly in the north and north-west of the country. Malaria, Chagas disease, leishmaniasis, schistosomiasis, dengue, leprosy, onchocerciasis and lymphatic filariasis are the NTDs with the highest prevalence rates.

The disease is also neglected by other spheres, such as the pharmaceutical industry and the health team. According to Gontijo (2003), ATL continues to be an extremely neglected disease, in other words, ignored by the big pharmaceutical conglomerates. Making matters worse, it is also little known by the general population, as well as by health professionals.

According to the Ministry of Health (2006), since the 1990s the Ministry of Health has reported an annual average of 32,000 new cases of ATL. Analysing the data for 2003, it was found that the North region reported 45% of cases, predominantly in the states of Para, Amazonas and Rondônia; the Northeast region, 26% of cases, mainly in Maranhão, Bahia and Ceara; the Centre-West region, 15% of cases, most frequently in Mato Grosso; the Southeast region, 11% of cases, predominantly in Minas Gerais; and the South region, 3.0%, with Paraná standing out.

It can be seen that proportionally the regions with the lowest HDI, such as the north-east and north, have the highest rates of cases, which are poorer regions and also where there may be greater negligence in combating the disease. On the other hand, the South, a region with a higher HDI, has fewer cases of the disease. According to Souza (2002), the 1996 Human Development Index (HDI) for Brazil was 0.830. The differences in HDI between geographical regions are marked, ranging from 0.608 in the Northeast to 0.860 in the South. The state with the lowest HDI is Piauí, with 0.534 and the state with the highest HDI is Rio Grande do Sul, with 0.869. This is due, among other factors, to the unequal investments/inputs allocated by the government by region in Brazil. As Carvalho (2002, p. 306) explains: "if we take the resources for health in Brazil, destined for assistance, as a whole, we will be certain of the inequity in their distribution". See the data below for the regions of Brazil (Chart 3).

Chart 3 - Federal health resources by region in Brazil (2000)

Region	**Per capita value RS**	**Comparison with Brazil average**
North	45,17	17.53% less
North-East	55,95	Minus 6.75%
South East	68,70	6% more
South	68,14	5.44% more
Centre-West	59,96	Minus 2.74 %

Source: Carvalho, (2002).

The number of ATL cases in Brazil has increased, particularly since 1985, with the Northeast and North regions having the majority of notifications. As ATL persists in areas that have suffered intense anthropisation, there is a need for permanent assessments to improve the treatment and prevention of this disease (LIMA et al, 2007).

However, despite being unknown, the disease is considered by the WHO to be one of the most important diseases. According to França (2009), the disease is considered by the World Health Organisation to be one of the most important endemic infectious and parasitic diseases. The number of cases in Brazil is growing, with a dual epidemiological profile, expressed by the maintenance of cases from old outbreaks or areas close to them and the appearance of epidemic outbreaks associated with factors such as the accelerated expansion of agricultural frontiers, the establishment of mining sites, the construction of roads and the process of invasion on the outskirts of cities.

In South America, only Chile and Uruguay have not registered any cases. The World Health Organisation considers Leishmaniasis to be one of the six most important infectious diseases. Due to its high level of detection and ability to produce deformities, it is classified as a neglected disease, due to the limited resources invested in diagnosis, treatment and control and its high association with the low-income population (WHO, 2011; BRAZIL, 2007; CDC, 2011).

ATL is found throughout Brazil. According to Basano & Camargo (2004), several Brazilian studies point to the occurrence of ATL and its vectors throughout Brazil, but with different incidence coefficients. It should be emphasised that the occurrence of the peri-urban transmission profile is related to the lack of basic sanitation, the precarious economic situation, the migration of the population to the outskirts of cities, inadequate building materials and living with wild or even domesticated animals, which serve as new reservoirs of the disease, together with the increase in the rat population that is concentrated in the rubbish dumps of these areas.

As it is a disease of significance to the WHO and has a wide geographical distribution in Brazil, recognising the affected population is of the utmost importance in order to achieve efficient levels of control. According to Viana et al (2012), the WHO considers ATL to be one of the six most important infectious diseases, due to its high degree of detection and ability to produce deformities. Therefore, knowing the identity of the population affected by ATL in Brazil is of fundamental importance for establishing effective measures to control the disease.

4.1.1 The incidence of the disease in Montes Claros

After being asked about the evolution of the disease in Montes Claros, **all but one of the** collaborators considered **the increase in the incidence of ATL** and its urbanisation in the research area. Among the reasons that could explain urbanisation, they mentioned deforestation, migration, the construction of highways, the proximity of homes to the forest, forest invasion, the displacement of the vector, the difficulty the phlebotome has in finding nutrients, the lack of vector control, the lack of sanitary conditions, the lack of basic infrastructure, the lack of structure in homes and the practice of sports such as climbing, hiking and fishing.

Interviewee E8 explains:

"It*'s evolved, that's a fact!* It *used to be more rural, but now* it's *moved into the* city, it's very urbanised. This has happened because of deforestation, because the vector is a rural mosquito; and as the municipality *has expanded a lot, urbanisation has begun."*

The study region has the essential conditions for an increase in the number of ATL cases, which is why the incidence of the disease has actually been rising. According to Monteiro et al (2005), in the municipality of Montes Claros there is a characteristic area that is favourable for leishmaniasis cases. In the outlying areas, the majority of homes are extremely poor, with no rubbish collection or basic sanitation. Many of the inhabitants have low socioeconomic indicators and there is a high level of coexistence with domestic animals, which results in the agglomeration of organic matter, providing suitable conditions for the transmission of the disease.

The municipality of Montes Claros has systematised records of human cases of

ATL, totalling 446 cases from 2002 to 2010, according to epidemiological data provided by epidemiological surveillance. According to Brasil (2012), different Brazilian regions have been suffering from the urbanisation of leishmaniasis in recent decades, which has led to an increase in cases of leishmaniasis. In the state of Minas Gerais, according to data from the Ministry of Health, the number of reported cases of ATL increased from 1,116 cases in 2001 to 1,887 reported cases in 2010.

The lack of an effective basic sanitation system, inadequate rubbish collection, socio-economic conditions and migration are also factors that favour the increase in cases of the disease. For Basano & Camargo (2004), it should be emphasised that the occurrence of the peri-urban transmission profile is related to the lack of basic sanitation, the precarious economic situation, the migration of the population to the outskirts of cities, inadequate building materials and living with wild or even domesticated animals, which serve as new reservoirs of the disease, combined with the increase in the rat population that is concentrated in the rubbish dumps in these areas.

According to Brasil (2000), the generation of organic waste by humans and domestic animals and the inadequate packaging of food favours colonisation by reservoir commensals (marsupials and rodents), with high infection rates. Waste must therefore be properly disposed of to avoid attracting animals.

In a descriptive study carried out by Machado-Coelho et al (1999), in the municipality of Caratinga-MG, comparing urban and rural areas, where the lack of basic sanitation and the accumulation of rubbish were greater, more cases of ATL occurred, and indicated that the lack of basic sanitation and rubbish can attract ATL hosts to domestic environments, where they find shelter and food (apud SOUZA, 2007).

For Viana et al (2012), the situation of poverty and poor basic sanitation may be opening the way for a new and worrying model of disease transmission, with endemic characteristics, for which health units must be prepared.

It should be emphasised that the occurrence of the peri-urban transmission profile is based on the lack of basic sanitation, the precarious economic situation, the migration of the population to the outskirts of cities, inadequate building materials and living with wild or even domesticated animals that serve as new reservoirs of the disease, as well as the increase in the rat population that is concentrated in the rubbish dumps of these areas (BASANO & CAMARGO, 2004).

Man-made environmental changes are also a factor in the increase in the incidence of the disease. According to Oliveira (2006), environmental changes caused by human beings have a direct effect on public health, impacting on disease transmission cycles, transforming habitats and displacing diseases close to the peridomiciles surrounding the impacted areas.

The increase in ATL cases over the years is due to human actions on the environment, such as the destruction of native vegetation. These actions directly change the behaviour and habitat of both vectors and reservoirs, allowing species to be selected and adapt to the anthropic environment, partly explaining the persistence of leishmaniasis in domestic and peridomiciliary areas. In addition, the disorderly construction of domestic animal shelters in the peridomiciliary environment and the lack of minimum basic sanitation conditions are common conditions in rural areas and on the outskirts of urban centres (SOUZA, 2007).

The epidemiology of ATL in the Americas is complex, with variations in transmission cycles, reservoirs, vectors, clinical manifestations and response to therapy, as well as the species of Leishmania circulating in the same geographical area. ATL was predominantly an occupational disease, related to activities such as rubber extraction, military operations, road construction and agricultural development. The occupational presentation continues to be important, but widespread deforestation has led to an accelerated increase in the number of cases, changing the epidemiological aspects of the disease. In Brazil, for example, from

1980 to 2001, there was a 10-fold increase in the incidence of ATL in all states (BRASIL, 2007; WHO, 2010).

The fundamental risk factors related to zoonotic cutaneous leishmaniasis in various regions of the world are urbanisation, deforestation, the establishment of new settlements, the domestication of the transmission cycle and the development of agriculture, with the construction of dams for irrigation. In the south-eastern region of Brazil, this disease has a peri-domiciliary transmission character, especially due to the adaptation of the insect vector to modified natural environments, thus enabling the involvement of domestic animals (NEVES et al, 2011).

Environmental changes have led to the domestication of phlebotomines, inducing a new model of transmission of the disease, since there are increasing rates of notification of ATL cases in populations that would have less risk of acquiring the disease (SILVA, 2009).

Mestre and Fontes (2007) stated that heavy deforestation is one of the main reasons for epidemic outbreaks of leishmaniasis in large cities. Intensive investigations into the ecology of these phlebotomines should be part of routine public health service activity, especially in regions with endemic leishmaniasis.

Outbreaks have been recorded in the state of Minas Gerais since the middle of the last century and the vast majority of cases are related to deforestation activities, road construction and the founding of agricultural projects (MARTINS et al, 1956; FURTADO, 1966). Over the years, this situation has changed, with outbreaks being recorded in areas that have already been colonised (HERMETO et al, 1994; GONTIJO et al, 2002), as well as appearing in peri-urban areas of cities, as for example in the study by Mayrink et al, (1979), carried out in the city of Caratinga, Vale do Rio Doce-MG (apud SOUZA, 2007).

ATL was limited to labourers who went into the forest and was considered an occupational disease. In the 1950s, after intense forest destruction, ATL almost disappeared. A significant increase in the disease reappeared in the 1980s, with autochthonous cases, in new geographical areas and in the form of an endemic, on the outskirts of urban centres, affecting the elderly and children, classically more restricted to the domestic environment and its surroundings, which indicates anthropisation (SILVA et al, 2010).

According to the Ministry of Health (2007), the transmission of ATL occurs in areas of preserved forest or forest with some alteration, where there is human presence.

Silva et al (2010) also admits that ATL has shown an increase in the number of cases and an increase in its geographical occurrence over the last 20 years. It is currently found in all Brazilian states, under different epidemiological profiles and transmission patterns as a result of socio-environmental changes. Cyclical variations in the incidence of leishmaniasis would be intensely influenced by geographical and climatic factors, which are responsible for fluctuations in phlebotomine populations.

In recent years, the disease has undergone a process of urbanisation, related to various contributing factors such as deforestation, migration, environmental changes, malnutrition, extensive engineering projects and precarious basic sanitation and living conditions for the population, exposing them to a greater risk of infection (DANTAS-TORRES & BRANDÃO FILHO, 2006; ANTONIALLI et al., 2007; FELIPE,2009).

Another problem reported by the interviewees is the proximity of homes to forest areas. In a descriptive, case-control study carried out in Bolivia, Alcais et al. (1997), considering the environmental characteristics of the homes involved in the cases, found that the proximity of the homes to forest areas, and the patients' places of work and leisure near the forest, also influenced the risk of contracting the disease (apud SOUZA, 2007).

According to Silva and Gurgel (2011), land occupation for housing purposes, when unplanned, favours the formation of residential centres very close to forests, leaving residual patches of forest between the houses.

These authors also consider that deforestation is largely due to the increase in the number of houses that are re-entering the forest. Homes are being built in places where there used to be only forest, and some of these houses have no piped water or sanitary infrastructure, suggesting the low economic standard of this population.

Other interviewees reported that with forest encroachment, the phlebotomus mosquito is deprived of nutrients and emerges in the city. Ribeiro et al (2007), in a descriptive study carried out in the municipality of Teófilo Otoni, observed that the growing number of ATL cases was related to the ecological imbalance produced by deforestation and disorderly land occupation. Deforestation of forest areas leads to the migration of natural reservoirs (wild animals) of Leishmania spp. to other areas in search of new shelters. As a result, phlebotomine sandflies, which used to fulfil their needs by feeding on these animals, start looking for other sources of food, including humans who already live in the vicinity of these recently deforested areas or who migrate to these places.

The interviewees also mentioned the characteristics of the home's infrastructure and sanitation as variables in the risk of transmitting ATL. In the case-control study carried out by Armijos et al (1997) in Ecuador, individuals living in houses built with plant material or mud had a higher risk of developing ATL than those living in brick-built houses. According to the authors, these risks were possibly related to the presence of gaps and holes in this type of material, which would cause the vector to enter the home and serve as a shelter for it (apud SOUZA, 2007).

For Silva and Gurgel (2011), in a study of the analysis of the spatio-temporal distribution of the disease, based on notified cases, carried out in Rio de Janeiro, the precariousness of homes, the lack of doors and windows with insect screens is what probably favours the vector invasion of ATL, especially at night, when mosquitoes are attracted by the light inside the house. It was also observed that deforestation for new illegal housing developments is happening rapidly and uncontrolled in the area, as there is no demarcation of plots or infrastructure (water, electricity, sewage) in a region that is difficult to access. Everything indicates that more people are moving to this area, which has already registered a large number of cases of the disease.

Comparing the opinion of the interviewees with the opinion of the authors whose statements we have been presenting, we see that the interviewees are focused on the reasons for the urbanisation of ATL.

4.1.2 Diagnosis of the disease

When asked if they thought that health professionals were able to identify cases of ATL, the interviewees had two types of answers. **The majority of** interviewees **(8)** were of the opinion that professionals **don't know how to** diagnose cases of ATL, as interviewee E9 explained:

"Training for medical professionals is lacking and needs to improve. Their training also needs to improve. Doctors make a lot of mistakes, they still fall short in diagnosis and treatment."

On the other hand, of the seven interviewees who said that professionals are able to diagnose the disease, **two** of them warned against **not notifying cases**, as interviewee E11 said:

"Yes (they know how to identify them), *but many don't report the cases, which makes it difficult for epidemiological surveillance to act in endemic areas."*

It is important to remember that this idea of doctors not being able to identify the exact diagnosis was put forward by the collaborators in this investigation, who were mostly made up of nurses and nursing technicians and the epidemiological surveillance team. In this study, we only had a sample of one doctor, so this data refers to the perception of other technicians about medical diagnostic competence.

Early and effective diagnosis is important for curing leishmaniasis lesions and for understanding the disease. According to Pellissari et al (2011), in order to reduce the lethality of these diseases, early diagnosis of cases and timely treatment are essential.

According to the same authors, in order to sensitise health professionals to the importance of proper treatment of patients with leishmaniasis, some short-term measures should be taken, such as: dissemination in newsletters for professional associations, publication of technical notes, dissemination at congresses, among other means of communication. In the long term, wide-ranging distance learning courses could be organised, as well as local training courses in areas where it is more difficult to manage these patients.

According to the Ministry of Health (2009), in order to guarantee good care for patients with ATL, it is necessary to train the professionals who will make up the multi-professional team, from the basic health units (UBS), laboratory diagnostic support and referrals, in laboratory and clinical diagnosis and treatment. Preliminary data from Rondônia points to an average leishmaniasis lesion evolution time of around 15 months, thus characterising a long period between the onset of the lesion and diagnosis, caused in part by the lack of diagnostic capacity and the lack of technical training of health professionals (BASANO & CAMARGO, 2004).

According to the Ministry of Health (2009), the following are the doctor's duties: diagnose people with ATL at an early stage, in accordance with the guidelines contained in the Ministry of Health's booklet; forward the ATL notification form to the epidemiological surveillance sector; notify cases of ATL and fill in the investigation form; notify any suspected cases of adverse reactions to the drugs indicated for ATL to the municipal epidemiological surveillance, so that it can notify Anvisa; request that the patient return after the end of treatment to assess clinical cure; refer cases of mucosal leishmaniasis and diffuse cutaneous leishmaniasis to the reference unit, respecting local flows and remaining responsible for follow-up; send the competent sector weekly epidemiological information on ATL in the UBS area and analyse the data for possible interventions; provide home care, when necessary; contribute to and participate in continuing education activities for team members regarding prevention, treatment management, epidemiological surveillance and control of ATL; and collaborate in the management of supplies and equipment at the BHU relating to ATL control actions.

The doctor will carry out the diagnosis at the BHU itself with spontaneous demand from the patient, and in places where there is greater exposure to the vector. According to Brasil (2007), patients can be cared for through spontaneous demand at health units, active search for cases in areas of transmission, when indicated by epidemiological surveillance or the family health team, or in risk areas where it is difficult for the population to access health units.

In order to support ATL surveillance and monitoring actions in Brazil, a website was opened, "allowing access to up-to-date, consolidated epidemiological information and online interaction between the National Coordination of the ATL Control Programme, based at the Health Surveillance Secretariat of the Ministry of Health (SVS/MS), and the state and municipal coordinators of this programme" (SVS/MS, 2011, p.1).

According to the Ministry of Health (2007), the flow of information in the federal unit should follow the SINAN guidelines. Monitoring and evaluation of the information system should be the responsibility of the technical area responsible for ATL surveillance at the three levels of management (municipal, state and federal). The data on the registration and investigation of ATL cases must be solid, adding information by municipality, administrative region and federal unit. This data is indispensable for the construction of the necessary indicators, the epidemiological analysis of the disease and the monitoring and operational evaluation of PLWHA at each management level.

SINAN was developed in the early 1990s with the aim of collecting and processing data on notifiable diseases throughout the country, providing information for analysing the morbidity profile and thus contributing to decision-making at municipal, state and federal levels (BRITO, 1993). The conception of SINAN was guided by the standardisation of case definition concepts, the transmission of data, based on the hierarchical organisation of the three spheres of government, access to the database needed for epidemiological analysis and the possibility of rapid dissemination of the data generated, in the routine of the National Epidemiological Surveillance System of the SUS. In addition, the system should be used as the main source of information for studying the natural history of an illness or disease and estimating its intensity as a health problem in the population, detecting outbreaks or epidemics, as well as forming epidemiological hypotheses to be tested in specific trials (BARRAL, 2009).

Immediate notification of ATL is important so that it can be investigated quickly, and treatment recommended, followed up monthly for 3 months to assess clinical cure (BRASIL, 2009). The data collection instrument is the SINAN epidemiological form, which contains the essential elements to be collected in a routine investigation. All the fields on this form must be carefully filled in, even when the information is negative or ignored. Other items and observations should be included, according to the needs and peculiarities of each situation. The form for recording and investigating cases of ATL makes it possible to know and evaluate information at the municipal, state and national levels (BRASIL, 2010).

Other studies also suggest that doctors make mistakes when filling in the form, which can jeopardise their knowledge and the final result of the treatment. According to Lima et al (2007), the obstacles to evaluating care activities for patients with ATL are diverse and of various kinds, including, among others, the failure to record information in patients' medical records, information contained in medical records that differs from that on the notification form, difficulty understanding the writing in medical records and the small number of studies on evaluation focused on this disease. Work on the evaluation of health programmes and services in Brazil only began to be published in the second half of the 90s.

4.1.3 Control actions and their effectiveness

When asked about the development of actions to control the disease and what these actions might be, **seven** interviewees replied that their sector has **not** developed control actions, as interviewee E15 states, saying that in practice this has not happened:

> *"In practice, we don't see activities that prioritise the control of ATL".*

The interviewees who said that **there are** control actions **(7)** gave as examples of these actions the monitoring of cases and the ATL surveillance programme, of which the examples that best represent their opinion are:

> *"Yes, monitoring cases, from when the patient is affected by the disease until they are cured." (E8)*

> *"One measure that I think is very important for the control of ATL is the ATL surveillance programme, which aims to discover cases early in the population [ ]"...(E11)*

Two of these respondents also gave their opinion on the **effectiveness of these actions**, pointing to the zoonosis centre as a control measure carried out by the municipality, as interviewees E3 and E5 illustrate:

> *"... Zoonoses work on the basis of the methodology recommended by the Ministry of Health, and the Ministry of Health does not order the zoonoses centre to control ATL [...] It orders us to control visceral leishmaniasis [...]".*

> *"...the municipality has a zoonosis centre where they identify sick dogs*

and collect them[ ]...."

Only one interviewee was unable to answer this question. The employees who considered the control measures to be effective described surveillance as the early detection of cases or the monitoring of patients once they have been affected by the disease. We realise, therefore, that these actions are not disease control or preventive, but rather curative, leading us to reflect on the misuse of public resources, which are still tied to the curative model to the detriment of a preventive and control proposal. As for the zoonoses centre, which is the sector empowered to take control measures for vector-borne diseases such as ATL, it does not take action for tegumentary leishmaniasis, but only for visceral leishmaniasis.

One of the actions of the zoonoses sector, the euthanasia of animals with leishmaniasis, is not recognised by the Brazilian Ministry of Health as an effective method. According to Desjeux (2004), Funasa (1999) and Brasil (2007), the control of leishmaniasis is one of the WHO's priorities. Measures such as eliminating vectors with insecticides in the home and peridomicile, impregnated collars to prevent canine infection, as well as sacrificing dogs with leishmaniasis, have not had the expected impact.

The Ministry of Health does not indicate actions to control wild and synanthropic animals in regions endemic for ATL and in cases of domestic animals with ATL, euthanasia is only permitted when mucosal lesions and secondary infections cause the animal to suffer (LAINSON; SHAW, 1988; BRASIL, 2007).

In some studies, eliminating seropositive dogs from a region has not reduced the rate of infection in humans. These data suggest that, in these cases, eliminating dogs without controlling the vector is not enough to prevent the spread of infection. In addition to the aforementioned measures, educational activities are also carried out with the population, taking into account social and cultural aspects, to ensure the community's understanding and involvement in the various aspects of disease surveillance and control (BRASIL, 2006).

According to Gontijo et al (2004), although in theory control strategies may appear adequate, in practice the prevention of communicable diseases by biological vectors is quite complicated, even more so when associated with the existence of domestic and wild reservoirs and environmental aspects, including physical aspects of the use of inhabited space.

It is important to remember the importance of the epidemiological profile in identifying risk regions and improving control measures. According to Lima et al (2007), epidemiological indicators are essential for assessing the magnitude of the disease, providing information for planning health actions in order to control the disease.

According to the Ministry of Health (2009), ATL is an endemic that presents great diversity and constant changes in the epidemiological patterns of transmission, in view of the different species of vectors, reservoirs and etiological agents that, associated with man's action on the environment, make control actions difficult. Control strategies must be specific, according to the epidemiological situation of each locality and region, and it is of fundamental importance to know the largest number of suspected cases, identify the circulating etiological agent and the predominant vector, know the areas where transmission is occurring and reduce human-vector contact through specific measures.

The different epidemiological profiles of ATL suggest different transmission control measures.

Transmission in forest areas would be efficiently prevented by vaccination, but unfortunately this tool is not available for use by people exposed to the vector, so one option would be to rely on early diagnosis and efficient clinical treatment. According to Basano & Camargo (2004), in the form of pure or modified sylvatic transmission, control actions are more difficult or not applicable due to the zoonotic nature of the parasitosis. In this case, one could bet on an efficient and operational vaccine, whether or not it provides sterilising immunity. Despite the abundance of studies in this direction, and some optimistic results, this important tool is not expected to be available in the short term, and control of the endemic with this transmission profile remains problematic. In this case, the provision of an efficient health system for the diagnosis and clinical management of cases would be an alternative for reducing the damage caused by the endemic.

As for the transmission profile in urban areas, the control measures would be the elimination of the vector, good management by the epidemiological surveillance team and, perhaps the most difficult aspect to achieve in Brazil, would be to improve the population's quality of life, including humane basic sanitation conditions. Basano & Camargo (2004) state that with regard to the peri-urban transmission profile, in addition to anti-vector measures and an efficient epidemiological surveillance system, reducing transmission is closely related to improving the population's living conditions, a problem that is beyond the technical scope of the health area and currently represents yet another obstacle in the endemic control approach.

The Brazilian Ministry of Health also advocates simple measures to avoid exposure to the vector. According to the Ministry of Health's LTA control manual (2009), there are mechanical means of preventing LTA, through the use of mosquito nets, fine screens on doors and windows, the use of repellents, the use of long-sleeved shirts, long trousers, socks and shoes (which are difficult to apply in regions with hot and humid climates).

There is also the American Tegumentary Leishmaniasis Surveillance Programme (PV-LTA), which aims to diagnose and treat detected cases at an early stage in order to reduce the deformities caused by the disease.

The specific objectives of PLWHA are: to identify and monitor territorial units of epidemiological relevance; to investigate and characterise outbreaks; to monitor severe forms with mucous membrane destruction; to identify autochthonous cases early in areas considered to be non-endemic; to reduce the number of cases in areas of household transmission; to adopt relevant control measures, following epidemiological investigation, in areas of household transmission; to monitor adverse drug events (BRASIL, 2010).

Chemical control through the use of residual action insecticides is the vector control measure recommended within the scope of collective protection. This measure is directed only at the adult insect and aims to prevent or reduce contact between the transmitting insect and the human population in the home, consequently reducing the risk of transmission (BRASIL, 2009).

However, some authors have drawn attention to the possible inefficiency of controlling the disease in the face of an increase in the number of cases. According to Silva and Cunha (2007), tegumentary leishmaniasis remains endemic in Brazil and the challenge of controlling it is growing. The growing trend of ATL cases observed in Brazil and the expansion of transmission to previously unaffected areas raise doubts about the impact of the control measures currently being carried out by the Ministry of Health (ROMERO & BOELAERT, 2010).

In order to define the strategies and the need for control actions for each area of ATL to be worked on, the epidemiological aspects should be considered, as well as their determinants (BRASIL, 2006). In the area surveyed, there is an increasing rate of the disease every year and considering control measures to be important would be essential.

The diversity of agents, reservoirs, vectors and the epidemiological situation of ATL, combined with the still insufficient knowledge of various aspects, highlights the complexity of controlling this endemic disease (BRASIL, 2007). For this reason, the bodies responsible should be more attentive to the disease in the north of Minas Gerais.

4.2.5 Degree of participation in the discussion and definition of ATL control actions

As for the involvement of management in the discussion and definition of actions for the control of ATL, the analysis of the interviewees' discourse shows that the **majority of** interviewees are **not** in management positions. **Only three** interviewees held **managerial positions** and after being asked this question, interviewees E8 and 10 clarified their perspectives on the manager's actions:

> *"We recently organised a seminar on ATL and VL. It was in the auditorium of the Exhibition Centre. It was for doctors and health professionals."*

> *"It's the health coordinator who goes to the meetings. I've already taken part in a VL project, but I don't think I've ever taken part in an ATL project."*

The manager explains:

> *"I supervise all discussions and decisions".* (E9)

Analysing the interviews, it can be seen that only two of the interviewees say that they actually take part in the discussion and definition of actions to control ATL, while the other mentions that he has never taken part in the discussion of these actions.

It is important to start from the basic premise of conceptualising management. According to Brasil (2010), management is the activity and responsibility of directing a health system (municipal, state or national), by exercising functions of coordination, articulation, negotiation, planning, monitoring, control, evaluation and auditing. SUS managers are therefore the Municipal and State Health Secretaries and the Minister of Health, who represent the municipal, state and federal governments respectively.

The managers of the SUS are the representatives of each sphere of government appointed to carry out the functions of the Executive in health, namely: at national level, the Minister of Health; at state level, the Secretary of State for Health; and at municipal level, the Municipal Secretary for Health (BRASIL, 2009).

The municipal government is the one that evaluates practices and results in order to achieve a certain objective. According to Brasil (2010), the manager of the municipal system is responsible for controlling, evaluating and auditing health service providers (state or private) located in their municipality.

In the case of leishmaniasis, it is recommended that the directorate of the health surveillance sector should supply basic health units with the necessary supplies for patient care and vector control. According to the Brazilian Ministry of Health (2006), under the health policy in force in Brazil, the control of leishmaniasis is the responsibility of the Unified Health System, where the Municipal Health Secretariats, supported by the state health secretariats, should, in accordance with the guidelines of the national leishmaniasis programme of the health surveillance secretariat, be responsible for organising the basic network for patient care and instituting actions to combat the vector.

The Health Surveillance Secretariat (SVS) works to promote and disseminate the use of epidemiological methodology at all levels of the SUS. It aims to establish information and analysis systems that allow the country's health situation to be monitored and support the formulation, implementation and evaluation of actions to prevent and control diseases and illnesses, the definition of priorities and the organisation of health services and actions (BRASIL, 2007).

The aim of health surveillance is to permanently observe and analyse the population's health situation, articulating a set of actions designed to control determinants, risks and damage to the health of populations living in certain territories, guaranteeing comprehensive care, which includes both individual and collective approaches to health problems (BRASIL, 2009).

Epidemiological surveillance is the key sector that provides assistance to municipalities for the control of ATL. According to França (2009), the epidemiological surveillance of the Health Departments, together with the Vectors Division/Zoonoses Management/Directorate of Epidemiological Surveillance/SES, will advise the municipalities on the operationalisation of the measures established for the control of ATL, as well as their adaptation to each reality.

The purpose of epidemiological surveillance is to provide permanent technical guidance to those who are responsible for deciding on the implementation of actions to control diseases and illnesses, by making up-to-date information available on the occurrence of these diseases or illnesses, as well as their conditioning factors in a specific geographical area or population. Subsidiarily, epidemiological surveillance is an important tool for planning, organising and operating health services, as well as for regulating related technical activities (BRASIL, 2007).

In addition, in 2007 the National Notifiable Diseases System (SINAN) was created, using information systems, which is yet another method aimed at supporting the surveillance and inspection of ATL in Brazil. According to Elkhoury et *al (2007),* in recent years SUS managers have been evaluating the quality of data and information, due to its importance in defining public policies, planning and decision-making, among other things. The information systems available have proved to be important tools, especially when they are related to each other and when data is analysed jointly, with the aim of complementing and expanding knowledge about diseases and illnesses of interest to public health.

4.2.6 Evaluation of control actions by basic health units (BHUs)

We tried to find out what the interviewees thought of the primary care Basic Health Units (UBS's) in the fight against and control of ATL, and we found that the answers were **more** directed towards **Unsatisfactory (9)**, as interviewee E6 illustrates:

"Health professionals themselves lack awareness and knowledge."

Only **four** interviewees considered the actions of the health units to be **Satisfactory**, explaining this alternative by the action of surveillance and assistance, as shown by interviewee E8:

> *"Very important work is being done in this regard, in relation to surveillance and assistance."*

Two interviewees were unable to answer this question and this finding suggests that the UBS's are not prepared to diagnose and treat patients with ATL. According to Viana et al (2012), the Montes Claros region is endemic for ATL, which is why health centres should be prepared to diagnose and treat the disease.

Basano & Camargo (2004) also share this opinion, stating that the lack of preparation of health centres for diagnosing ATL is undoubtedly a major obstacle to an early approach to the patient. Normally, most health centres are not trained to carry out parasite testing and/or do not have the antigen to carry out the diagnostic test. According to the Brazilian Ministry of Health (2009), Primary Health Care Teams should carry out surveillance and control actions for tegumentary leishmaniasis, with the priority of diagnosing and treating detected cases early, with the aim of reducing deformities caused by the disease; monitoring adverse events to medicines and working in conjunction with the municipality's health surveillance team.

According to the Ministry of Health (2009), in order to structure and organise diagnostic and treatment services, as well as to guarantee the quality of care for patients with ATL, it is necessary to identify the health units and multi-professional teams that will assist the patients; define the laboratory diagnostic support and the professional from the basic health unit or reference unit who will carry out the parasitological examination.

The Ministry of Health recommends that UBS's should be trained to treat patients and, when necessary, refer them to referral centres, which in our study is the University Hospital. Actions aimed at the early diagnosis and appropriate treatment of ATL cases are the responsibility of the Municipal Health Secretariats (SMS), with the support of the State Health Secretariats (SES). To this end, it is necessary to organise the basic health network to suspect, assist, monitor and, when indicated, refer patients with suspected ATL to outpatient or hospital referral units. All referred patients will be co-responsible for the Primary Health Care Teams in their area of residence, and these teams must accompany and support patients during treatment at referral units and monitor counter-referrals for post-treatment follow-up. The conditions for early diagnosis and treatment must therefore be provided, as well as establishing the flow of referrals and counter-referrals.

The Ministry of Health (2009) also makes it a priority for UBS's to establish a flow of referrals and counter-referrals for clinical and laboratory diagnosis and treatment; to implement or improve the flow of information of interest to surveillance and care; and to regularly evaluate and publicise the actions carried out by the services, as well as the epidemiological situation of ATL.

There is still a way to measure *the* quality of UBSs. According to Neves *et al* (2011), the municipalisation of health actions and services increasingly requires the use of evaluation methods to support changes in guidelines and strategies that will contribute to improving the health system. The State Health Secretariats and the Ministry of Health, in the area of controlling diseases of interest to Sanitary Dermatology, have been assessing the impact of actions according to the *American Tegumentary Leishmaniasis Control Manual*, using a set of epidemiological and operational indicators that make it possible to determine the trend and extent of the endemic, as well as measuring the condition of the activities carried out by the municipalities' BHUs.

4.2.7 Involvement of health workers in ATL control

When asked if the municipality's health professionals promoted control measures for ATL, **most of** the interviewees **(7)** answered **No**, as the following quote shows:

"No! The involvement is more for visceral leishmaniasis, we hardly hear about tegumentary *leishmaniasis*, maybe people don't even know the seriousness of the disease[ ]... There's a lack of involvement." (E15)

Six interviewees reported that **there is control**, as interviewee 11 explains:

> *"I do* (have control), *an example is the sanitary agents and zoonosis control. "*

Two interviewees were unable to answer this question and, again, those who did were referring to Visceral Leishmaniasis and not Tegumentary Leishmaniasis. According to Lima *et al* (2007), UBS professionals may not be aware of the indications in the American Tegumentary Leishmaniasis Control Manual.

The Ministry of Health (2007), among other control measures, recommends training health professionals to improve the fight against and control of ATL. According to the same source, the approach to peri-domiciliary transmission centres, practising sanitation conditions to prevent the accumulation of rubbish and debris that can attract rodents and small mammals, together with improvements in housing conditions should be carried out. In addition to these measures, there should be more training for health professionals at all levels.

Basano and Camargo (2004) also state that the increased indicators of ATL detection in the municipalities may be related to the lack of information on measures to prevent American tegumentary leishmaniasis, which are probably not publicised to the community by the UBS teams. Such measures could significantly reduce the population of phlebotomine sandflies in the peridomicile and household, helping to reduce the risk of transmission, especially among rural dwellers. In addition, improving basic sanitation and housing conditions, together with training UBS professionals to apply educational measures, could favour a reduction in the number of people with the disease and the misuse of medication.

Health workers play an important role in capturing the vector for entomological research. According to Brasil (2009), considering the diversity of species of phlebotomine vectors, it is important to carry out entomological surveys with the aim of knowing their presence and distribution in areas with and without ATL transmission, especially in the home and peridomiciliary environment. To this end, it is also a priority for the UBS team, through the Community Health Agents, to collaborate in entomological surveillance activities (capture of the phlebotomus mosquito), identifying suitable places to install traps in their area of coverage, as well as helping the technicians to install and remove the traps. Endemic disease control agents can also help with this work.

Home visits and providing information are the responsibility of UBS professionals. According to Brasil (2007), in the regions with the highest number of ATL cases, the Family Health Programme teams can play an important role in actively searching for cases and adopting educational activities with the community. In areas with a peri-urban profile or with old settlements, an attempt should be made to reduce vector contact through the use of residual insecticides, the use of individual protection measures such as mosquito nets, fine screens on windows and doors, repellents and clothing that protects exposed areas and a minimum distance of 200 to 300 metres from houses in relation to the forest.

The following are duties common to all primary care/family health professionals: to participate in the planning, management and evaluation of the actions developed by the Primary Care Team in tackling ATL; to define strategies in conjunction with the Leishmaniasis Programme; to ensure follow-up and continuity of care for both suspected cases and those with confirmed diagnosis of ATL; to carry out active searches for suspected cases; provide continuous care, in conjunction with the other levels of care, with a view to longitudinal care; plan and develop educational and community mobilisation actions in relation to the control of ATL in their area of coverage, in conjunction with epidemiological surveillance and stimulate intersectoral actions that contribute to the control of ATL.

According to the Ministry of Health (2009), the duties of endemic disease control agents and community health agents are: identify suspected cases of ATL, by means of signs and symptoms, and refer them to the UBS's for investigation, diagnosis and treatment; work in households and other community spaces, informing their residents and other citizens in the area covered by the Basic Health Unit about the disease, its symptoms and risks, the transmitting agent and prevention measures; inspect the home, peridomicile and other locations in the territory accompanied by the residents and/or citizens to identify places that are breeding grounds for the vectors; advising the population on the removal of organic matter (rubbish, food waste, animal droppings) that could become breeding grounds for vectors; advising the community on the use of individual and family protection measures to prevent ATL; promoting meetings with the community to mobilise them for ATL prevention and control actions, as well as raising awareness of the importance of all households being as clean as possible, so that vector control is indirectly achieved.

Finally, Barral (2009) states that the measures taken by health professionals to control ATL must be flexible and distinct, based on the particular epidemiological characteristics, combined with a basic health system that is capable of early diagnosis and appropriate treatment.

4.2.8 Strategies used to control ATL

When asked about the strategies used to control ATL, **four** employees said that **no** information actions **are carried out** and **six** said that the information given is **insufficient**, as there are only control strategies for Visceral Leishmaniasis, as stated by the interviewees below:

"The *few strategies are not aimed at ATL, only visceral." (E4)*

"We have publicity, talks, seminars and events for people in public squares. But we have control for VL, not for ATL." (E8)

A smaller proportion of employees (**only 4**) gave other answers such as **Sufficient,** as explained by the interviewees below:

"*We sometimes use standers, lectures, talks in pubs, churches,* where there is a crowd of people who need to receive this *information and in the face of a requested demand. "* (E3)

"Through training, informing people how to identify the disease." (E5)

Analysing the discourse of these four interviewees allows us to say that the strategies used are essentially banner exhibitions, talks and informal conversations in social spaces.

Only one interviewee was unable to answer this question, and once again, a large proportion of the interviewees pointed to information measures and strategies only for VL. The Ministry of Health assigns education measures to both VL and ATL. According to the Brazilian Ministry of Health (2006-2007), in Brazil, the VL and ATL manuals include health education activities and determine their inclusion in all services that develop leishmaniasis control measures, calling for the effective involvement of multi-institutional and multidisciplinary teams, with the aim of articulating the work in various service-providing units. It can be deduced that the control strategies are not adequate for the population of Montes Claros.

The population's lack of knowledge is an aggravating factor in controlling the disease. According to Sampaio *et al* (2009), the epidemiological importance of leishmaniasis in public health demands the development and cheapening of drugs to treat it. Several factors make it difficult to control these diseases: the lack of a vaccine, the wide variety of leishmania and phlebotomus species, the population's lack of knowledge and prevention of the disease, among others.

It's painful to think that low-cost measures to stimulate information could reverse the increase in ATL. According to Teodoro et *al* (2007), through cheap alternatives and practical measures that can be added to the habits of people living in high-risk areas, the incidence of leishmaniasis can be reduced. This means that the most effective prevention and control of these vectors requires public evaluation and the effectiveness of health efforts and community participation in their implementation.

It is hoped that ways of publicising the disease will have to be implemented in order to raise awareness and sensitise the population to the factors that determine the development of ATL cases, through health education teams to guide prevention and clarify the forms of transmission (UCHOA et al, 2004).

These disease-causing vectors, especially leishmaniasis, are linked to poor socio-economic and sanitary conditions, which is why control measures must be systematically achieved. It is essential to define public health policies that can resolve existing distortions and inequalities in health standards. These must go beyond current actions and find new alternatives, such as better access to education, better housing, higher income and nutrition, basic sanitation and environmental protection. Health education can offer people simple knowledge of breeding sites, vector locations and can result in a significant reduction in the incidence of the disease. As is true for all diseases of public health importance, basic and general knowledge must be widely disseminated (KISHORE et *al,* 2006). We realise that we need to step up the pace in order to successfully achieve information strategies on ATL in the municipality of Montes Claros.

The Brazilian Ministry of Health (2009) also stresses that the results of entomological research into the mosquitoes that transmit ATL should be disseminated to guide the population in adopting measures to prevent and combat the insect vectors.

The actions of the Municipal Health Department also include raising awareness among the population about the responsibility of each resident in the fight against leishmaniasis (BARRAL, 2009). For this reason, the population must be efficiently and actively orientated.

Furthermore, cases may be underreported due to lack of knowledge of the cutaneous lesion of ATL. According to Nunes et al (2008), due to the population's lack of knowledge about the disease and difficulties in accessing health centres, it is possible that cases are still being underreported, especially in rural areas. As a result, the number of cases may be higher than reported.

4.2.9 The decentralisation of services

Regarding the aspect of recognising the department responsible for coordinating, managing and carrying out ATL control actions, the question was asked whether decentralisation of ATL control in the municipality of Montes Claros has been implemented. **Five** of the interviewees believe that **decentralisation** is already in place, while **four** of the interviewees believe that ATL control services are **centralised** and that decentralisation is not being implemented in Montes Claros, and most of the interviewees **(6) were unable to answer** this question. Of the interviewees who mentioned decentralisation of services, the answers were in the direction of health units notifying cases and guiding patients, as interviewees E13 and E15 illustrate:

> "[ ]...*I believe so, just the fact that the basic units have the* autonomy to notify and refer is already a step towards this *decentralisation.* "
>
> *"Yes* (decentralised), *because the patient arrives at any health unit and reports what they're feeling and is given initial guidance at the unit itself, and is then referred to the referral hospital, which is the HU."*

Of the four interviewees who believe that the service is **centralised**, there was **unanimity** in pointing to the reference centre for leishmaniasis in Montes Claros, the **University Hospital,** as the only place where diagnosis, treatment and control of ATL is carried out, as stated by interviewees E10 and E8:

"It's all done right there in the HU."

"The centralisation was requested by the University Hospital; the doctors there are specialists, it's the reference centre; because some prescriptions come without adjustments from other places, because of the amount of serum infused; it doesn't authorise the medication. That's why we leave everything there."

The decentralisation of health services began in Brazil around the 2000s, with the aim of improving and perfecting service inputs and expenditure, to increase the autonomy of the municipality to receive financial resources and distribute them better, and the formation of UBSs to better meet spontaneous demand.

For a better understanding of the way in which services are organised in Brazil, we will give you a brief history. Law No. 1,920 of 25 July 1953 split the Ministry of Education and Health into two: the Ministry of Health and the Ministry of Education and Culture. The Ministry of Health became part of the National Health Department (DNS).

Three years after the creation of the Ministry of Health, Decree 2.743 created the National Department of Rural Endemic Diseases (DNERu), which was tasked with "organising and executing research services and promoting the fight against malaria, leishmaniasis, Chagas disease, plague, brucellosis, yellow fever, schistosomiasis, hookworm disease, filariasis, hydatidosis, endemic goitre, yaws, trachoma and other endemic diseases existing in the country, the research and fight of which were especially assigned to it...". This decree also established the National Institute of Rural Endemics (INERu), whose remit was to "carry out research and studies into the endemics indicated with the aim of increasing knowledge of them and improving prophylactic methods to combat them" (SILVEIRA & JUNIOR, 2011 p.3).

The National Epidemiological Surveillance System (SNVE) was structured in 1975, with the enactment of Law No. 6.259, regulated by Presidential Decree No. 78.231. Due to the limited coverage of health services at the time it was established and in line with the epidemiological situation prevailing at the time of its creation, the SNVE operated only on communicable diseases, and was solely the responsibility of the federal and state governments. The municipalities played no role in the management of the health system (BRASIL, 2007).

The implementation of the decentralisation action led to changes in the internal arrangement of the National Health Foundation (FNS), especially with regard to the coordination and fulfilment of vector-borne disease control actions, which until then had been the responsibility of the Operations Department (DEOPE) and which, from 1999, passed to the National Epidemiology Centre (CENEPI), which incorporated the management of the national health surveillance system as its responsibilities. These responsibilities fundamentally involved the national coordination of Health Surveillance actions, especially those activities that establish national or regional simultaneity, such as technical standards, the management of epidemiological information systems and the provision of resources and equipment (SILVEIRA & JÚNIOR, 2011).

The 1990s saw a process of regulation of the decentralised management of public policies in many areas such as health, education, social assistance, among others, with the inclusion of society's participation, through management, in their formulation and control. These councils are now considered to be the most expressive links in the emergence of a new system of public action in the local sphere, characterised by the opening up of new patterns of interaction between government and society in the management of public policies (SANTOS JÚNIOR, 2001).

According to Rocha (2009), the Management Councils thus constitute the new institutional format provided for in the articles of the 1988 Federal Constitution, which establish participation in various areas: in *health,* as "community participation" (art. 198, item II); in *social assistance,* as "participation of the population", through representative organisations, in the formulation of social policies and control, at all levels of government (art. 204, item II); and in *education,* as "democratic management of public education" (art. 206, item VI).

According to Silveira & Júnior (2011), the process of decentralising disease prevention and control actions in Brazil began in 2000, with the publication of Ordinance M.S 1399 of December 2002, which deliberated and regulated the responsibilities of each of the fields of government in this area and established the construction of funding, on a fund-by-fund basis.

The process of implementing decentralised management in health surveillance, among other aspects, was conditioned by a solution to the financing of these actions, which had previously been carried out through direct execution or agreements between FUNASA and states and/or municipalities, which generally covered specific disease control programmes. With the publication of Ordinance GM/MS No. 1,399, in December 1999, the logic of financing changed, establishing a fund-to-fund transfer of the Health Surveillance Financial Ceiling (TFVS) to states and municipalities certified to carry out health surveillance actions. This had a positive effect on disease prevention and control, as the municipalities began to take on a large part of the health surveillance actions, and the states became responsible for coordinating and supervising the process, as well as carrying out the actions. The regulation of this process was updated by Ordinance GM/MS No. 1,172, published on 17 June 2004 (BRASIL, 2007).

This has led to the emergence of new initiatives for the democratic management of public policies, with the introduction of institutional reforms aimed at strengthening the independence of municipalities and establishing new ways of organising local power, linked to the creation of partnerships between public authorities and organised sectors of society (ROCHA, 2009).

In 2003, the Ministry of Health reorganised the area of epidemiology and disease control with the extinction of the National Epidemiology Centre (CENEPI) and the creation of the *Health Surveillance Secretariat.* This came to bring together all the attributions of CENEPI and the programmes that were part of the now defunct Secretariat for Health Policies (BRASIL, 2007).

Endemic disease control is another important step in the process of decentralising health actions within the SUS. It is a new strategy for reducing and even eliminating endemic diseases in Brazil. Epidemiology and disease control actions have been decentralised from the FNS to the states and municipalities (BRASIL, 2002).

However, these decentralisation initiatives still face obstacles in terms of their effective implementation. According to Rocha (2009), the current dynamics of the shared management model involve the democratic nature of participatory processes. Although deliberation is more democratic than in previous models, because it is submitted to a greater number of people, it is a democratic deliberation from the point of view of formal democracy.

Therefore, this model of participatory and decentralised management in Brazil has faced major barriers, since the centralising and authoritarian tradition that has always marked Brazilian territory has imposed on government agencies a pattern of management that is completely independent of society and subsidised by both the dictates of the bureaucracy and the interests of those in power. This is why it is essential to reaffirm the importance of management councils as an essentially political space where organised citizens can interact with representatives of the powers that be (ROCHA, 2009).

The Health Councils are collegiate bodies made up of representatives from the government, service providers, health professionals and users, with the latter holding 50 per cent of the membership. These collegiate bodies are permanent and deliberative in nature, and work to formulate strategies and monitor the implementation of health policy at the corresponding level. The Councils comprise a network of Municipal Health Councils, a State Health Council in each state and a National Health Council. The implementation of this system, particularly with regard to the decentralisation process and the definition of the role of each sphere of government, is conditioned by and must face at least three demands: the marked inequalities that exist in the country, the challenges in the area of health and the characteristics of Brazilian federalism (SOUZA, 2002). The decentralisation process therefore appears to be far from complete.

4.2.10 Human, material and monetary resources for the control of ATL

We asked the participants in the study whether the human and material resources involved in the control of ATL are sufficient, and the **majority of** interviewees **(11)** responded by indicating the **Insufficiency** of these resources, as explained by the interviewees:

"I need printed material, more training, I really think there's a lack of posters in the area and information in the media." (E1)

"There is a lack of human resources to increase education and vehicles..." (E9)

"Everything is missing, there's a lack of equipment and medication." (E12)

Only two employees replied that it was **Sufficient**, emphasising that:

"I think so. There's good work in the area." (E 5)

"In the institution where I work, yes, there is enough material to control the disease. I don't know about primary care, but I believe there is, because the resources come along with other funds offered." (E15)

Only two interviewees were unable to answer this question and it is presumed that the lack of human and material resources is another factor that implies that ATL control is not functional in the municipality surveyed. According to Dantas-Torres & Brandão-Filho (2006) and Felipe (2009), the fact that the application of the recommended measures has not been achieving satisfactory results is accompanied by problems such as the scarcity of resources and the current lack of infrastructure in health services, especially in relation to the diagnosis of leishmaniasis infection, which has made the current control measures inefficient in many Brazilian states, where leishmaniasis remains yet another neglected disease.

Considering the complexity of the actions to be developed in the region, with cases of tegumentary leishmaniasis, it is essential for planning to analyse the need for professionals, by type and level of training, as well as the infrastructure (physical space, equipment, etc.) (BRASIL, 2007).

Current methods of controlling leishmaniasis are limited to the peridomestic environment and have proved inadequate (Alexander et al.,1995; Sessa et al.,1994). The control methodologies advocated for another population distribution situation have not kept up with the demand generated by the rate of growth and the increasing occupation of areas at risk of the disease. Associated with this, a relatively high percentage of subclinical forms have been detected in individuals living in some risk areas, which makes it difficult to determine these areas (Marzochi and Marzochi,1994). Furthermore, the lack of financial resources for prevention and control activities has hindered technical and scientific development and the training of human resources in this area (apud MASSA & MARQUES,1996).

In order to achieve the condition of care for patients with ATL, it is necessary to supply health units with the materials and supplies needed for diagnosis and treatment.

According to the Ministry of Health (2009), the routine activities of UBSs and Health Surveillance should be developed with a view to making the principles and guidelines of universal access and comprehensive care viable, according to health needs, where the use of epidemiology to establish priorities, allocate resources and guide programmes is of fundamental importance.

According to the Ministry of Health, it is recommended that funds be efficiently allocated to the purchase of vehicles and equipment for endemic disease control, but the interviewees reported the absence of these resources. According to the Brazilian Ministry of Health (2007), in addition to the TFVS funding modality, the secretariat also has an Investment Plan for the purchase of vehicles and other equipment with a view to helping strengthen the management of the Health Surveillance System in the areas of Epidemiological Surveillance and the Control of Communicable and Non-Communicable Diseases/Agravities, Environmental Health Surveillance and Health Situation Analysis in the state and municipal health spheres.

There is a lack of human and material resources for the effective ongoing control of ATL. According to Mendes (2002), because primary care is seamless, care and cure jobs are likely to be longer, more extensive and more varied. More extensive types of resources must often be applied.

Finally, the employees were asked if they were aware of the amount allocated by the government to control ATL in the municipality of Montes Claros. **Almost all of** the interviewees **were unable to answer** this question and according to the only interviewee (9) who did answer the question, the money allocated by the government is not specifically for the control of ATL:

"There are no specific resources for the control of ATL. In a recent project for VL, we got 300,000.00. The resources are general health resources, for combating all communicable diseases, and leishmaniasis is included in all of them[...]They're waking up now for ATL. The number of cases is increasing a lot, but so far there's nothing specific."

The demarcation of a health region, according to established criteria, includes an analysis of the population's needs in terms of existing resources. These resources interfere with the risk of various diseases or illnesses occurring (BARRAL, 2009). There are no specific resources for controlling ATL.

Efficient resources are needed to actively combat leishmaniasis. According to Barral (2009), the Plan to Combat Leishmaniasis includes the training of health professionals and an amount allocated by the government to combat it. The funds earmarked for the payment of the various health care actions provided between municipalities are allocated in advance by the manager who demands these services to the municipality where the provider is based. This municipality incorporates the funds into its financial ceiling. Budgeting is based on agreed and integrated programming between managers (BRASIL, online: http://conselho.saude.gov.br/legislacao/nobsus96.htm#4).

The Basic Operational Standard of the SUS - NOB-SUS/96, in its item 14, already provides for the transfer of financial resources, fund by fund, to states and municipalities, to cover the cost of epidemiological actions and the control of diseases/illnesses, formalising the creation and operation of local epidemiological surveillance systems, with differentiated resources for each area, according to the development of these systems, which will be conferred by the results valuation index of NOB/SUS/96. (CENEPI/FNS, on line: http://www.ebah.com.br/enfermagem).

In addition to transfers from the FNS, state and municipal funds receive contributions from their own budgets. Some states transfer their own resources to municipal health funds, according to rules defined at state level. The federal level is still responsible for the largest share of SUS funding, although the participation of municipalities has been growing over the last ten years and there is a prospect that the share of state resources in funding the system will increase significantly as a result of the approval of EC-29 (BRASIL, 2009). The decentralisation of health services has better subsidised the results of budgetary action for the municipalities.

According to the Brazilian Ministry of Health (2009), payment to health service providers is made by the level of government responsible for their management. The tendency is for municipalities to take on more and more responsibility for the relationship with service providers, as they qualify for the decentralised management conditions of the system. The standard in force (NOAS-SUS 01/01) establishes two conditions for municipal management: (a) Full Management of Expanded Primary Care, whereby the municipality qualifies to receive a defined amount, on a per capita basis, for the funding of primary care actions, and (b) Full Management of the Municipal System, whereby the municipality receives the total federal funds programmed for the cost of care in its territory. It should be clarified that funding on a per capita basis does not exempt the manager from having to feed the outpatient information system, the output of which will serve as input for future negotiations on the allocation of financial resources.

The process of implementing decentralised management in health surveillance, among other aspects, was conditioned by the solution to the financing of these actions, previously carried out through direct execution or agreements between FUNASA and states and/or municipalities, which generally included specific disease control programmes (BRASIL, 2007).

Until 1997, there was no subdivision of the funds transferred to states and municipalities, which began to occur in March 1998 with the publication of Ordinance No. 2121/GM, which established the Basic Care Floor (PAB) and opened up the funds for financing Basic Care and for financing Medium and High Complexity Outpatient Care.

Each municipality's PAB, which is calculated based on a per capita value, is automatically transferred from the FNS to the Municipal Health Funds, changing the previous form of financing by providing services and moving to a logic of transferring resources, due to the municipality's commitment to assume health responsibility for this level of care (BRASIL, 2009). The PAB for the municipality of Montes Claros in 2012 was 7,485,722.49 Reais.

With the publication of Ordinance GM/MS No. 1,399 of December 1999, the logic of financing changed, establishing a fund-to-fund transfer of the TFVS to certified states and municipalities for the development of health surveillance actions. This allowed for greater rationality and effectiveness in the prevention and control of diseases, as the municipalities began to take on a large part of the health surveillance actions, and the states became responsible for coordinating and supervising the process, as well as carrying out the actions on a supplementary or complementary basis (BRASIL, 2007).

The TFVS is exclusively intended to finance health surveillance actions. The funds are transferred in monthly instalments directly from the FNS to the health funds of the states and municipalities certified to manage these actions (BRASIL, 2006). The fight against ATL should follow a specific budget system for fighting the disease. In the current year, 2012, 2,105,768.51 Reais were transferred to health surveillance (promotion and general care of all communicable and non-communicable diseases). The categories and subcategories that emerged from the interviews per interviewee are presented below, in a table that aims to summarise the analysis carried out (Table 4).

Table 4 - Summary of categories and sub-categories by interviewee

Category	Subcategory/interviewee (n°)
• Interviewees' knowledge of ATL • Is ATL a priority disease?	-Yes (El-15). -Yes (El-5; E7-8; Ell-15); -No(E6; E9-10).
- The incidence of the disease in Montes Claros	- Evolved and urbanised (EI-14) - It hasn't evolved and it hasn't urbanised (E15).
- Diagnosis of the disease	- Professionals don't know how to diagnose (E2-4; E6; E8-9 and E14-15). - Professionals know how to diagnose (E1; E5; E7 and E10-13).
- Control actions and their effectiveness	- Ineffective (El-3; E6; E13-15)

	- Effective (E4-5; E7-9; EI 1-12) - Couldn't answer (E10)
- Degree of participation in the discussion and definition of ATL control actions	-Not part of the management (El-7; EI 1-15). - Participates effectively (E8-9). -Never participated in a discussion on LTA (E10)
- Evaluation of control actions by basic units	- They are not satisfactory (El-4; E6; E8; Eli; E13 and E15). -Satisfactory (E5; E7 and E9-10). -Couldn't answer (E12 and E14).
- Involvement of health workers in ATL control	- No (El-3; E10; E12-13 and E15). -Yes (El; E5; E7-9 and Eli). - Couldn't answer (E6 and EI4).
- Information actions/strategies on ATL	- It's not done (El; E2; EI 1 and E12). - Insufficient (E4; E7-9; E13 and E15). - Sufficient (E3; E5; E10 and E14). - I couldn't answer (E6). - Exhibitions, talks and informal conversations.
- Decentralisation of services	- Decentralised (El, E5, Eli, E13 and E15). - Centralised (E3; E8-9 and E10). -Couldn't answer (E2; E4; E6; E7; E12 and E14).
• Human and material resources for LTA control • Monetary resources for LTA control	- Insufficient (E1; E3-4; E6-12 and E14). - Sufficient (E5 and E15). - Couldn't answer (E2 and E6). - Couldn't answer (E1-8; E10-15). - Non-specific monetary resource for LTA (E9).

CHAPTER 5

CONCLUSIONS

After a detailed analysis of the results and discussion, we are now in a position to draw up a set of conclusions, taking into account the objectives initially proposed and the research questions that guided this study.

This study has provided an insight into public policies in relation to the control of American Tegumentary Leishmaniasis (ATL) in the municipality of Montes Claros and, in view of all the conclusions reached during the course of this work, some final considerations should be made on the subject. The findings of this study point to relevant aspects for reflection on the health actions that are proposed and implemented.

Researching the health services offered for ATL shows that this disease is a health priority in most cases in the municipality. However, it can be deduced that there are cases that seem to suggest some negligence in controlling this disease, with greater priority being given to other illnesses such as meningitis, dengue and hepatitis.

Almost all the interviewees agree with the official statistics on the incidence of the disease and its evolution, indicating that it has been increasing and urbanising. They therefore have a correct perception of the reality of this disease in the region. The interviewees also point to a number of factors that have contributed to the urbanisation of the disease, such as the marked deforestation in the Montes Claros region, constant migration, the practice of sports and leisure activities in regions close to forests and the construction of homes and houses adjacent to the forest, which are referred to in the literature consulted.

The interviewees' opinion favours the lack of competence among health professionals to diagnose the disease, and they also point to the existence of underreporting of cases.

It is also clear that the actions to control ATL in the municipality are carried out through surveillance, with the early discovery of cases and/or the monitoring of patients. In this way, we realise that these actions are not disease control or preventive, but rather curative, raising questions about the archaic way in which curative resources are used, rather than disease control and prevention. The zoonoses centre was also mentioned by some collaborators, but reports indicate that zoonoses are controlled only for visceral leishmaniasis.

According to the interviewees, most of the basic health units are inefficient, showing that they are not prepared to diagnose and treat patients, and that health professionals may not be aware of the control measures for ATL.

It is clear from the interviews that the strategies used to control ATL are limited to actions to disseminate information about the disease, but these are insufficient for the needs of the population. In some cases, even information sessions on the disease are non-existent.

As for the degree of participation in the discussion and definition of ATL control actions, most of the interviewees who hold management positions actually take part in these actions and the other employee has never taken part in the discussion of these actions, mentioning them only for visceral leishmaniasis. In other words, this participation is not part of the experience of all the managers who work in this area.

The group of interviewees is practically split down the middle when it comes to their opinion on decentralisation, with those who believe that there is decentralisation of disease control services and those who believe that this is not the case and that they are still centralised, which shows that the implementation of decentralisation is not yet complete and that there is still a long way to go in this direction, despite the fact that decentralisation was put into practice in the 2000s as a national health policy in Brazil. It was also noted that the human and material resources involved in controlling the disease are considered insufficient and that the funds allocated to ATL are not specifically earmarked for this disease. The interviewees identified a number of missing resources, in addition to human resources, such as printed material, posters, access to the most up-to-date information, equipment, medicines and transport.

The interviewees are therefore aware of the deficiencies in public health services for ATL and the need to make significant adjustments and improvements, both in direct patient care and in the way the network of services for ATL sufferers is organised, structured and run. It is therefore hoped that municipal managers, the community and professionals in the field will seek ways to transform this reality.

It can therefore be concluded that there is no effective control of ATL in the municipality of Montes Claros, and there is still much to be done in order to achieve effective control of the disease in our region.

In view of these conclusions and the problems identified, we propose a set of suggestions for improving the effectiveness and efficiency of ATL control actions, which we will describe below:

- Increasing the dissemination of information on ways of preventing, treating and controlling the disease, so that the population becomes aware of the disease and knowledgeable about the agents of development and ways of preventing ATL.

- The creation of more effective public policies aimed at combating misinformation, especially by primary health care, which is the great and main ally of programmes to combat ATL and disseminate this information;

- Providing more human resources to increase education and vehicles that increase their mobility and bring them closer to the people;

- Diversify the strategies for controlling the disease, in addition to information such as early discovery of cases and adequate sanitary conditions;

- Encourage capacity-building and training programmes for health professionals specialising in disease control actions;

- Activating services in primary health care units for ATL, as one of the possibilities for improving patient care, since clinical reception in neighbourhoods close to residents is a powerful instrument that links early and appropriate diagnosis and treatment;
- Creation of a Leishmaniasis reference centre.

CHAPTER 6

REFERENCES

Abbagnano, N. (2003). Dictionary of Philosophy. São Paulo: Martins Fontes.

Almeida, E., Castro, C., & Vieira, C. (2002). Health districts: conception and organisation. In: Health and citizenship. For municipal health managers. Institute for Health Development. Faculty of Public Health, University of São Paulo. Ministry of Health. Núcleo de Assistência Médico- Hospitalar-NAMH/FSP.

Almeida, P., Giovanella, L., Mendonça, M., & Escorel, S. (2010). Challenges to the coordination of health care: strategies for integration between levels of care in large urban centres. *Cad. Saúde Pública,* 26 (2).

Almeida, O.S. & Santos, J.B. (2011). Advances in the treatment of new world tegumentary leishmaniasis in the last ten years: a systematic review of the literature. An. *Bras. Dermatol.,* 86 (3).

Amato, V.S. (2006). *Treatment of American tegumentary leishmaniasis.* Leishmaniasis Outpatient Department of the Infectious and Parasitic Diseases Clinic. Hospital das Clínicas-(26). Faculty of Medicine, University of São Paulo.

Amatuzzi, M.M. (2003). *Subjectivity and its research.* Memorandum, 10, 93-97.

Andrade, C.C. (2007). The client's experience in the psychotherapeutic process: a phenomenological study in Gestalt Therapy. *Rev. abordagem gestalt.,* 13, (1)17-168.

Andrade, E.I.G., Acúrcio, F., Cherchiglia, M.L., Belisário, S.A., Júnior, A.A.G., Szuster, D.A.C., Faleiros, D.R., Teixeira, H.V., Silva, G.D., & Taveira, T.S. (2007). Research and scientific production in health economics in Brazil. Rev. Adm. Pública, 41(2), 211-235.

Antonialli, S.A.C., Torres, T.G., Filho, A.C.P., & Tolezano, J.E. (2007). Spatial analysis of American visceral leishmaniasis in Mato Grosso do Sul, central Brazil. *Journal of infection,*54, 509-514.

Assis, M.M.A., Villa, T.C.S., & Nascimento, M.A.A. (2003). Access to health services: a possibility to be built in practice. *Ciênc. saúde coletiva,* 8 (3), 815-823.

Barata, R.A., Paz, G.F., Bastos, M.C., Andrade, R.C.O., Barros, D.C.M., Silva, F.O.L., Michalsky, E.M., Pinheiro, A.C., & Dias, E.S. (2011). Phlebotomine sandflies (Diptera: Psychodidae) in Governador Valadares, an area of transmission of American tegumentary leishmaniasis in the State of Minas Gerais, Brazil. Rev. Soc. *Bras. Med. Trop.,* 2 (3), 136139.

Barral, N.M. (2009). Immunological aspects of diffuse cutaneous leishmaniasis. *Gaz. Méd. Bahia,79,* 35-39.

Basano, S.A. & Camargo, L.M.A. (2004). American tegumentary leishmaniasis: History, Epidemiology and Perspectives for Control. *Rev. bras. epidemiol.,*7(3), 328-337.

Bonacim, C.A.G. & Araújo, A.M.P. (2011). Evaluation of the economic and financial performance of health services: the effects of operational policies in the hospital sector. *Ciênc. saúde coletiva,* 16 (1), 1055-1068.

Bosi, M.L.M., & Affonso, K.C. (1998). Citizenship, popular participation and health: with the word, the users of the Public Services Network. *Cadernos de Saúde Pública*, *14*(2), 355-365.

Botelho, A.C.C. (2006). American tegumentary leishmaniasis: histopathological and immunophenotypical changes. *Rev.Soc.Bras.Med.Trop.*, 39(1),14-21.

Brazil. Federal Official Gazette (1990). Law no. 8.080. Provides for the conditions for the promotion, protection and recovery of health, the organisation and operation of the corresponding services and makes other provisions.

Brazil. Ministry of Health (1991). Basic Operational Standard - NOB 01/91. Brasília.

Brazil. Ministry of Health (1995). *Constitution of the Federative Republic of Brazil*: promulgated on 5th October 1988. Org. Juarez de Oliveira. (11ª edition). São Paulo: Saraiva.

Brazil. National Congress (1996). Law 9.311, of 24 October 1996. Federal Official Gazette.

Brazil. Ministry of Health (1998). *American Tegumentary Leishmaniasis in Brazil (Ferida Brava)*. Information booklet for health workers. Brasilia: National Health Foundation.

Brazil. Civil House (2000). Constitutional Amendment 29, of 13 September 2000. Federal Official Gazette.

Brazil, Ministry of Health (2000). Manual de Controlo da Leishmaniose Tegumentar Americana /Organisation: Gerência Técnica de Doenças Transmitidas por Vetores e Antropozoonoses. Epidemiological Surveillance Coordination - National Epidemiology Centre. National Health Foundation. Ministry of Health. Brasília.62 p.

Brazil. Ministry of Health (2001). Operational Standard for Health Care. NOAS-SUS 01/01. Brasília.

Brazil. Ministry of Health (2005). Health Surveillance Secretariat. *Guide to epidemiological surveillance.* Secretaria de Vigilância em Saúde. (6. ed.). Brasília 146p.

Brazil. Ministry of Health (2006). *National Agenda of Health Research Priorities.* Basic Health Texts (2.ed.) Series B. Brasília: Ministry of Health Publishing House.

Brazil. Ministry of Health (2006). Ordinance GM/MS 399 of 22 February 2006.

Federal Official Gazette.

Brazil. Ministry of Health (2006). Health Surveillance Secretariat. Department of Epidemiological Surveillance. *Atlas of American tegumentary leishmaniasis: clinical and differential diagnosis.* Brasília. Editora do Ministério da Saúde,136 p.

Brazil. Ministry of Health (2006). Health Surveillance Secretariat. *National health surveillance system: situation report:* Minas Gerais

Gerais / Ministério da Saúde, Secretaria de Vigilância em Saúde,Brasília, (2ª .ed.), 24p.

Brazil. Ministry of Health (2007) Health Surveillance Secretariat. Department of Epidemiological Surveillance. Manual de Vigilância da Leishmaniose Tegumentar Americana, Brasília, (2nd ed.),182p.

Brazil, Ministry of Health (2007). Health Surveillance Secretariat. Report on activities carried out in 2006. Synthesis. [on line]. Available: www.portal.saúde.gov.br.

Brazil, Ministry of Health (2009). Health Surveillance Secretariat. *Health Surveillance.* [on line]. Available: www.saude.gov.br / svs.

Brazil. Ministry of Health (2009). Health Care Secretariat. *Health surveillance : zoonoses* / Ministry of Health, Secretariat of Health Care, Department of Primary Care. -Brasília : Ministry of Health.Cadernos de Atenção Básica, (1st ed.), 22, 224p.

Brazil. Ministry of Health (2009). Health Surveillance Secretariat. Health Surveillance Management Support Directorate. *Health surveillance management manual* / Health *Surveillance Management* Support Directorate. Brasília. 80p.

Brazil, Ministry of Health. *Norma Operacional Básica do SUS (2010).* [onlin e].

Available: http://conselho. saude.gov.br/legislação/nobsus96.htm#4

Borges, J.M. (2009). O choque de gestão na saúde de Minas Gerais. Organised by Antônio Jorge de Souza Marques. Belo Horizonte. Minas Gerais State Department of Health. 324 p.

Camossa, A.C.A., Telarolli, J.R. & Machado, M.L.T. (2012). The nutritionist's theoretical-practical practice in the family health strategy: social representations of team professionals. Revista de Nutrição,25(1), 89-106.

Carvalheiro, J.R. (2008). *Epidemics on a global scale and in Brazil.* Estud. av. 22(64), 7-17.

Carvalho, G.C.M. (2002). O financiamento público federal do sistema único de saúde *1988-2001* [master's thesis]. São Paulo (SP): School of Public Health, University of São Paulo.

Castro, S.S., Lefèvre, F.L., Cavalcanti A., & Cesar, C.L.G. (2011). Accessibility to health services by people with disabilities. *Revista de Saúde Pública*, *45*(1), 99-105.

Centres for Disease Control (1968). *Comprehensive plan for epidemiological surveillance*. Atlanta, Ga. National Epidemiology Centre, National Health Fund. [on line]. Available at: http: //www. ebah.com.br/enfermagem

Companhia Energética de Minas Gerais (2006). Environmental Assessment and Licensing Management. Camargos HPP, Volume I, *Environmental Control Report and Plan.* Belo Horizonte, 243p.

National Council of Municipal Health Secretaries (CONASEMS) (2007). Incomplete agenda, management guidelines and thesis at CONARES *Jornal do CONASEMS,v.* 6.

Costa, C.R.C. (2002). Decentralisation, financing and regulation: the reform of the Public Health System in Brazil during the 1990s. *Rev. Sociol. Polít.*,18:49-71.

Cunha, A.B.O. & Silva, L.M.V. (2010). Accessibility to health services in a municipality in the State of Bahia, Brazil, under full system management. *Cad. Saúde Pública,* 26 (4), 725-737.

Dantas, T.F. & Brandão, F.S.P. (2006). Geographical expansion of visceral leishmaniasis in the state of Pernambuco. *Journal of the Brazilian Society of Tropical Medicine,* 39(4), 352-356.

Desjeux, P. (2004). Leishmaniasis: current situation and new perspectives. Comparative Immunology, Microbilogy and Infectious Diseases, 27, (5), 305-318.

Dias, E.S., França, S.J.C., Silva, J.C, Monteiro, E.M., Paula, K.M., Gonçalvez, C.M. & Barata R.A. (2007). Phlebotomines (Diptera: Psychodidae) from an outbreak of tegumentary leishmaniasis in the state of Minas Gerais. *Rev. Soc. Bras. Med. Trop,* 40 (1), 49-52.

Elkhoury, A.N.S., Carmo, E.H., Gomes, M. L., & Mota, E. (2007). Analysis of visceral leishmaniasis records by the capture-recapture method. *Revista de Saúde Pública,* 41(6), 931-937.

Escorel, S, Giovanella, L, Mendonça, MHM, & Senna, MCM. (2007). The Family Health Programme and the construction of a new model for primary care in Brazil. Rev. *Panam. SaludPública,* 41(6),164-76.

Felipe, I.M.A. (2009). Spatial distribution of Leishmania (L) chagasi infection and seroprevalence in an endemic area, municipality of Raposa-MA, Dissertation [master's degree], Federal University of Maranhão.

Flick, U. (2004). *An introduction to qualitative research;* transl. Sandra Netz. (2[a] ed-312p.), Porto Alegre, Bookman.

Freese, E.M. de C., Fábio, L., Gonçalvez. F.R., Silva, J.A.M., & Lima, M.E.F. (1998). The process of epidemiological transition and social inequity: the case of Pernambuco. *Rev. Associação Saúde Pública Piauí,*1 (2), 107119.

National Health Foundation (FUNASA) (1999). Temporal evolution of notifiable diseases in Brazil from 1980 to 1988. *Epidemiological Bulletin,* Special Ed.

Furtado, T., Aleixo, J. & Lopes, C. F., (1966). Outbreak of American tegumentary leishmaniasis in Minas Gerais. *Cad.Saúde Pública,* 70 (12), 259266.

Furtado, T. (1994). *American tegumentary leishmaniasis.* In: Machado Pinto J(ed), Infectious diseases with dermatological manifestations. Editora Médica e Científica Ltda, p.319-328.

Gadelha, C.A.G., Machado, C.V., Lima L.D. de & Baptista, T.W.de F. (2011). Health and territorialisation from a development perspective. *Ciênc. saúde coletiva,* 16 (6), 3003-3016.

Gasparotto, L.P.R., Reis, C.CI., Ramos, L.R., & Santos, J.F.Q. (2012). Self-assessment of posture by elderly people with and without thoracic hyperkyphosis. *Ciênc. saúde coletiva,* 17 (3), 717-722.

Gil, A.C. (2007). *Methods and Techniques of Social Research* (5th ed.), 8th reprint, São Paulo, Atlas.

Gomes, F.M. & Silva, M.G.C. (2011). *coletiva,* 16 (1). The Family Health Programme as a primary care strategy: a reality in Juazeiro do Norte. *Ciênc. Saúde,16* (1), 893-902.

Gomes, A.C., & Neves, V.L.F.C. (1998). Strategy and perspectives for the control of tegumentary leishmaniasis in the State of São Paulo. *Revista da Sociedade Brasileira de Medicina Tropical,* 31(6), 549-552.

Gontijo, B. & Carvalho, M.L.R. (2003). American tegumentary leishmaniasis.

Revista da Sociedade Brasileira de Medicina Tropical, 36(1),71-80.

Gontijo C.M.F., Melo M.N. (2004). Visceral Leishmaniasis in Brazil: Current Situation, Challenges and Perspectives. *Rev.Bras.Epidemiol.,7,(3')* 338349.

Gontijo, T.L., Xavier, C.C., & Freitas, M.I. F. (2012). Evaluation of the implementation of the Kangaroo Method by managers, professionals and mothers of newborns. *Cadernos de Saúde Pública, 28*(5), 935-944.

González Rey, F. (2002). *Qualitative research in psychology: paths and challenges.* São Paulo: Pioneira.

González Rey, F. (2005). *Qualitative research and subjectivity.* São Paulo, Thomson.

Habicht, J.P., Victora, C.G., Vaughan, J.P. (1999). Evaluation designs for adequacy, plausibility and probability of public health programme performance and impact. *International Journal of Epidemiology,* 28(1), 1018.

Hartz, Z. (1997). *Evaluation in health.* Rio de Janeiro: Fiocruz.

Holanda, A. (2006). Questions about qualitative research and phenomenological research. *Psychological Analysis,* 24 (3), 363-372.

Hotez, P.J., Molyneux, D.H., Fenwick, A., Savioli, L., Takeuchi, T. (2008). The neglected tropical diseases of Latin America and the Caribbean: a review of disease burden and distribution and a roadmap for control and elimination. Plos Negl.trop.Dis, *New Engl.J.Med,* 2:e300.

Hotez, P.J. & Molyneux, D.H. (2007). Control of neglected tropical diseases. *New Engl.J.Med.,* 2 (7), 1018-1027.

Japiassu, H. & Marcondes, D. (2006). *Basic Dictionary of Philosophy.* Rio de Janeiro: Jorge Zahar.

Jesus, W.L.A., & Assis, M.M.A. (2010). Systematic review on the concept of access in health services: contributions from planning. *Ciência & Saúde Coletiva,* 15(1), 161-170.

Júnior, J.S.C., Fernandes, M.I.M, Jorge, S.M., Maciel, L.M.Z., Santos, J.L.F., Júnior, AlS.C., Passador, C.S., & Camelo, S.H.H. (2011). Health economic evaluation: neonatal screening for galactosemia. Cad. Saúde Pública, 27 (4),666-676.

Junqueira, T.S., Cotta, R.M.M., Gomes, R.C., Silveira, S.F.R., Siqueira, R., Pinheiro, T.M.M.. & Sampaio,R.F. (2010). Labour relations in the context of the municipalisation of health management and the dilemmas of the expansion/precarisation of work relationship in the context of the SUS. Cad. Saúde Pública, 26 (5), 918-928.

Kishore, K., Kumar, V., Kesari, S., Dinesh, D.S., Kumar, A.J., Das P., Bhattacharya, S.K. (2006) .Vector control in leishmaniasis. *Indiana J Med Res,* 123 (3), 467-472.

Lainson, R. & Shaw, J.J. (1988). New world Leishmaniasis - The *Neotropical Leishmania species.* In: Topley;Wilson. Microbiology and Microbial Infections, (9th ed.). London: Ed.Feg Cox.

Leite, M.E., Batista, R.P., & Clemente, C.M.S. (2010). Spontaneous segregation in the city of Montes claros/MG. *Electronic journal of the geography course.* Campus Jataí.Universidade Federal de Goías.

Leite, M.E. & Pereira, A.M. (2005). Territorial expansion and the spaces of poverty in the city of Montes Claros. *Proceedings of the 10th Meeting of Latin American Geographers*. University of São Paulo.

Lima, M.V.N., Oliveira, R.Z., Lima, A. P., Felix, M.L.O., Silveira, T.G.V., Rossi, R.M., & Teodoro, U. (2007). Care of patients with American tegumentary leishmaniasis: evaluation in the health services of

municipalities in the north-west of the state of Paraná, Brazil. *Cadernos de Saúde Pública,* 23(12), 2938-2948.

Lima, A.P., Minelli, L., Teodoro, U., & Comunello, E. (2002). Distribution of tegumentary leishmaniasis by orbital remote sensing images in the State of Paraná, Southern Brazil. *Anais Brasileiros de Dermatologia,* 77, (6), 681-692.

Lindoso, J.A.L., & Lindoso, A.AB.P. (2009). Neglected tropical diseases in Brazil. *Revista do Instituto de Medicina Tropical de São Paulo,* 51(5), 247253.

Maywald, P.G., Machado,M.I., CostaJ.M., & Gonçalves M.R.F. (1996).Tegumentary and visceral leishmaniasis and canine Chagas disease in municipalities of the Triângulo Mineiro and Alto Paranaíba, Minas Gerais, Brazil. *Cad. Saúde Pública,* 12 (3), 321-328.

Marques, R.M. (1999). The financing of the Brazilian public health system. CEPAL/GTZ Project. *Reformas a los sistemas de salud en América Latina.* Santiago de Chile.

Martinez, J., Martineau, T. (2002). Human resources in the health sector: an international perspective [on line]. Available at: http: //www.healthsistemsrc .org

Martins, J. & Bicudo, M. (2005). *Qualitative research in Psychology: foundations and basic resources.* São Paulo: Centauro.

Marzochi, M.C.A., & Marzochi, K.B.F. (1994). Tegumentary and visceral leishmaniases in Brazil: emerging anthropozoonosis and possibilities for their control. *Cadernos de Saúde Pública, 10*(Suppl. 2), S359-S375.

Massa, J.L. & Marques, C.C.A. (1996). Analysis of the occurrence of American tegumentary leishmaniasis using images obtained by orbital remote sensing in an urban locality in the Southeast region of Brazil. *Rev. Saúde Pública,* 30(5), 433-

437.

Mathers, C.D., Ezzati, M. & Lopes, A.D. (2007). Measuring the burden of neglected tropical diseases: the global burden of disease framework. *PLoS Negl. trop. Dis,* (1), p.114,.

Mendes, E.V. (2002). *Primary health care in the SUS.* Fortaleza: Ceará School of Public Health.

Mestre, G.L.C., Fontes, C.J.F. (2007). The expansion of the visceral leishmaniasis epidemic in the state of Mato Grosso, 1998-2005. Rev. *Soc. Bras. Med. Trop.,* 40, (3), 42-48.

Minayo, M.C.S. (2006). *The Challenge of Knowledge: Qualitative Research in Health* (9th ed.), São Paulo: Hucitec.

Minas Faz Ciência (2012). *American Tegumentary Leishmaniasis.* [on line]. Available at: revista.fapemig.br

Montes Claros. City Hall (2010). *Epidemiological Surveillance.* Municipal Health Department.

Monteiro, E.M., França, J.C., Costa, R.T., Costa, D.C., Barata, R.A., Paula, E.V., Machado, G.L.L., Rocha, M.F., Fortes,C.L., Dias, E.S. (2005). Visceral leishmaniasis: Study of phlebotomines and canine infection in Montes Claros, Minas Gerais. *Rev. Soc. Bras. Med. Trop.,* 38,(4), 147152.

Mora, J. F. (2001). *Dictionary of Philosophy.* São Paulo: Martins Fontes.

Moreira, V. (2004). Merleau-Ponty's phenomenological method as a critical tool in psychopathology research. *Psicologia: Reflexão e Crítica,* 17 (3), 447-456.

Murback, N.D.N., Filho, G.H., Nakazato, K.R.O., Nascimento, R.A.F., & Dorval, M.E.M.C. (2011). American tegumentary leishmaniasis: clinical, epidemiological and laboratory study carried out at the University Hospital of Campo Grande, Mato Grosso do Sul, Brazil, *An. Bras. Dermatol.,86* (1).

Netto, E.M. (1990). Long-term follow-up of patients with Leishmania (viannia) braziliensis infection and treated with Glucantime®. *Trans. R. Soc .Trop. Med. Hyg.,* 84 (3), 367-370.

Neves, D. (2001). *Parasitologia Humana.* (11. ed.) São Paulo: Atheneu.

Neves, J. (1983). *Diagnosis and treatment of infectious and parasitic diseases.* (2. ed.) Rio de Janeiro: Guanabara Koogan.

Nobrega, C.B.C., Hoffmann, R.H.S., Pereira, A.C. , & Meneghim, M.C. (2010). Financing the health sector: a recent retrospective with an approach to dentistry. *Ciênc. saúde coletiva,15* (1), 1763-1772.

Nogueira, R.P. (2006). Problems of management and regulation of labour in the SUS. Serviço Social e Sociedade, *Revista Serviço Social e Sociedade*, 87,p.1-14.p.12.

Nunes, A.G., Paula, E.V., Teodoro, R., Prata, A. & Silva, M.L. *et al.* (2006). Epidemiological aspects of American tegumentary leishmaniasis

in Varzelândia, Minas Gerais, Brazil. *Cad. Saúde Pública, 22 (6),* 12431247.

Oliveira, M.V.A.S.C. (2001). *New endemic disease control policies: decentralisation as hope for a change in the epidemiological profile.* Mimeo.

Oliveira, A.G.R.C., Souza, E.C.F. (1998). Health in Brazil: trajectories of an assistance policy. *Social dentistry: selected texts.* Federal University of Rio Grande do Norte, p.114-121.

Oliveira, W.W. (2011). The importance of health promotion actions carried out by nurses in the family health team. Master's dissertation. Federal University of Minas Gerais.

Oliveira, F.A.S., Heukelbach, J.M., Rômulo C.S., Ariza, L., Ramos, J., Alberto N., & Gomide, M. (2006). Large dams and their impact on public health: upstream effects. *Caderno de Saúde Coletiva ,14,* (4), 575596.

Oliveira, F.A.S., & Heukelbach, J. (2006). Large dams and their impact on public health: upstream effects .*Caderno de Saúde Coletiva,14,* (4), 575-596.

World Health Organisation (WHO) (2009). Leishmaniasis. Burden of disease. [on line]. Available: http://www.who. int/leishmaniasis/burden.en/

Pan American Health Organisation (PAHO). (2002). *Basic health indicators in Brazil*: concepts and applications. Ripsa.

Pan American Health Organisation (PAHO-WHO) (1998). World Health Organisation. Health in Brazil. Brasilia.

Pan American Health Organisation (1994). Leishmaniasis in the Americas, PAHO, v.1, p.8-13. (Boletin Epidemiologico, 15).

World Health Organisation (WHO) (1990). [on line]. Available at http//www. who.int

Paim, J.S., & Teixeira, C.F. (2006). Health policy, planning and management: a review of the state of the art. Rev *Saude Publica, 6, (2)* 73-78.

Pelissari, D.M,Cechinel, M.P., Souza,M.L., & Júnior, F.E.F.L (2011). Treatment of Visceral Leishmaniasis and American Tegumentary Leishmaniasis in Brazil. *Epidemiol. Serv. Saúde.* 20 (1).

Penna, G.O., Domingues, C.M.A.S, Siqueira, J., J.B., Elkhoury, A.N.S.M, Cechinel, M.P., Grossi, M.A.F., Gomes, M.L.S., Sena, J.M., Pereira, G.F.M., Lima, J., Francisco, E.F., Segatto, T.C.V., Melo, F. C., Rosa, F.M., Silva, M.M., & Nicolau, R. A. (2011). Dermatological diseases of compulsory notification in Brazil. *Anais Brasileiros de Dermatologia,* 86(5), 865-877.

Pimenta, D.N., Leandro, A., & Schall, V.T. (2007). The aesthetics of the grotesque and audiovisual production for health education: segregation or empathy? The case of leishmaniasis in Brazil. *Cad. Saúde Pública,* 23,(5), 1161-1171.

Municipality of Montes Claros-MG-Brazil (2012). The city of Montes Claros. [on line]. Available at https.www.montesclaros.gov.br

United Nations Development Programme (UNDP) (2000).Atlas of Human Development.

Interagency Network of Information for Health (RIPSA).(2002). *Basic health indicators in Brazil.* Brasilia: Pan American Health Organisation (PAHO).

Rey, L. (1991). *Parasitology.* Rio de Janeiro: Guanabara Koogan.

Rey, L. (2002). *Bases of Medical Parasitology* (2.ed.) Rio de Janeiro: Guanabara Koogan.

Roncalli, A.G. (2000). The organisation of demand in public oral health services: universality, equity and integrality in collective oral health. Araçatuba (SP): Araçatuba School of Dentistry. Master's thesis. Paulista State University.

Rocha, R. (2009). Decentralised and participatory management. *Revista Pós Ciências Sociais,* 1 (11), 1-5.Saraiva, L., Lopes, J.S., Oliveira, G.B.M., Batista, F.A., Falcão, A.L., & Andrade, J.D. (2006). Study of phlebotomines (Diptera: Psychodidae) in an area of American tegumentary leishmaniasis in the municipalities of Alto Caparaó and Caparaó, State of Minas Gerais. *Journal of the Brazilian Society of Tropical Medicine,* 39(1), 5663.

Health, Directorate General of Health (DSIA) (2001). Glossary of Concepts for the Production of Health Statistics, *Information Circular,* no. 19.

Rio de Janeiro State Health Department. *Zoonosis control centre.* [on line]. Available at: http: //www. saude. rio .rj .gov.br

Municipal Secretariat for Economic Development, Tourism, Science and Technology (2008). [on line] Available at: http.montesclaros.gov.br,accessed on 31/08/12 at 10:12).

Silva, E.M. (2001). Social Representations of American Tegumentary Leishmaniasis: an ethnographic study. Dissertation[master's degree] in Public Health.Recife.

Silva, L.M.R. & Cunha, P.R. (2007). The urbanisation of American tegumentary leishmaniasis in the municipality of Campinas - São Paulo (SP) and region: magnitude of the problem and challenges. An *Bras Dermatol.,* 82 (6), 5159.

Silva, A.E.P. & Gurgel, H.C. (2011). American tegumentary leishmaniasis and its socio-environmental relations in the municipality of Ubatuba-SP. *Revista Franco Brasileira de Geografia,* 13 , 1-45.

Silva, N.S., & Muniz, V.D. (2009). Epidemiology of American tegumentary leishmaniasis in the state of Acre, Brazilian Amazon. *Cad. Saude Pública,* 25(6), 1325-36.

Silva, A.F., Latorre, M.R.D.O., & Galati, E.A.B. (2010). Factors Related to the Occurrence of American Tegumentary Leishmaniasis in the Ribeira Valley. *Rev. da sociedade brasileira de medicina tropical,* 43 (1), 46-51.

Souza, J.T. (2008). Information and communication technologies in maths degree courses. Master's dissertation. University of São Paulo.

Souza, Y.B. (2007). American tegumentary leishmaniasis in the municipality of Ilhéus-BA: characterisation of human cases and associated risk factors. Dissertation [master's degree], Federal University of Viçosa.

Souza, R.R. (2002). The *Brazilian public health system.* International Seminar. Trends and Challenges of Health Systems in the Americas. São Paulo, Brazil.

Souza, R.R. (2003). Reducing regional inequalities in the allocation of federal health resources. *Ciência & Saúde Coletiva,* 8(2), 449-460.

Tanaka, O.Y. & Tamaki, E.M. (2012). The role of evaluation for decision-making in health services management. *Ciênc. saúde coletiva,* 17 (4), 821-828.

Teodoro, U., Santos, D.R., Santos, A.R., Oliveira, O., Poiani, L.P., Kuhl, J.B., Lonardoni, M.V.C., Silveira, T.G.V., Monteiro, W.M., & Neitzke, H.C. (2007). Evaluation of phlebotomine control measures in northern Paraná State, Brazil. *Cad. Saúde Pública,* 23,(11) 2597-2604.

Tomasi, E., Facchini, L.A., Thumé, E., Piccini, R.X., Osorio, A., Silveira, D.S., Siqueira, F.V., Teixeira, V.A., Dilélio, A.S., & Maia, M.F.S. (2011). Characteristics of the use of primary health care services in the South and Northeast regions of Brazil: differences by model of care. *Ciência & Saúde Coletiva,* 16(11), 4395-4404

Tonelli, E. & Freire, L.M.S. (2000). *Infectious Diseases in Childhood and Adolescence* (2. ed.), Rio de Janeiro: Guanabara Koogan.

Uchôa, C.M., Serra, C.M.B., Magalhães, C.M., Silva, R.M.M., Figliuolo, L.P.,Leal, C.A., Madeira, M.F. (2004). Health education: teaching

on American tegumentary leishmaniasis. Cad. Saúde Pública, 20(4), 935-41.

Federal University of Rio Grande do Sul. Norms and techniques in research involving human beings. [on line]. Available at: http://www.bioetica.ufrgs.br/res19696.htm

V argas, D.M., Arena, L.F.G.L., & Soncini, A.S.. (2010). Secular trend of height growth in Blumenau-Brazil and its association with the Human Development Index (HDI). Journal of the Brazilian Medical Association, 56(3), 304-308.

V iana, A.L.Á., Fausto, M.C.R., & Lima, L. D. (2003). Health Policy and Equity.

São Paulo em Perspectiva, 17(1), 58-68.

V iana, A.G., Souza, F.V., Paula, A.M.B., Silveira, M.F., & Botelho, A.C.C. (2012). Clinical and epidemiological aspects of American tegumentary leishmaniasis in Montes Claros, Minas Gerais. Rev. Med. Minas Gerais, 22(1), 1-128.

V idal, S.A., Samico, I.C., Frias, P.G., & Hartz, Z.M.A. (2011). Exploratory study of costs and consequences of prenatal care in the Family Health Programme. Revista de Saúde Pública, 45(3), 467-474.

V ilson, R. & Sande, A. (2004). Infectious diseases: diagnosis and treatment. Porto Alegre: Artmed.

World Health Organisation (WHO) (1978). United Children's Found (UNICEF). *Health for all.* Geneva: World Health Organisation.

World Health Organisation (WHO) (1981). *Health programme evaluation.* Geneva.

CHAPTER 7

Annexes

Annex 1

INTERVIEW SCRIPT

Evaluation of the effectiveness of ATL control policies in the municipality of Montes Claros
Group I - Characterisation of the interviewees

1 - Interviewee's gender: Female □ Male □

2 - Age:years

3 - Education: ___________________________

4 - Profession:___________________________
4.1 - Career category:
4.2 - How long have you been in your job?

Group II - Staff perceptions of ATL control policies

5 - Have you ever heard of LTA?

5.1 - If so, do you consider ATL to be a priority disease in the municipality?

5.2 - If not, why?

5.3 - Do you think that the sector has developed actions to control the disease?

5.3.1 - If so, which ones?

5.4 - With regard to the participation of managers in discussing and defining of actions to control ATL, how involved are you?

5.5 - Do you think that health professionals are able to identify cases of ATL?

5.6 - How do you rate the services offered by health centres? when it comes to fighting and controlling ATL?

5.7 - Has the decentralisation of ATL control in the Municipality of MOC been implemented?

5.7.1 - If so, do you think that decentralisation has made LTA control more effective?

5.7.1.1 - Why?

5.7.2 - If not, what are the operational barriers to administrative decentralisation?

5.8 - How do you think the incidence of the disease has evolved in the municipality of MOC?

5.8.1 - Why?

5.8.2 - Do you think the disease is urbanising?

6. In your opinion, have the health workers in the Municipality of MOC been involved in the work to control ATL?

6.1. If so, how?

6.2. Have information actions been carried out about the disease?

6.2.1 . If so, what strategies do you use?

6.2.2 - In your opinion, has there been any concern to adapt them to the characteristics of the community/population? Can you give us some examples?

7 - Do you know the amount of money allocated by the government to control ATL in the Municipality of MOC?

7.1 - If so, do you consider this government budget (transfer) for the control and fight against ATL to be sufficient? Please justify your opinion.

7.2 - Have the funds earmarked for this purpose been well spent? Justify your opinion.

7.3 - Are the human and material resources involved in LTA control sufficient?

7.2.1 - If not, what do you think is missing?

8 - Is there anything you'd like to add about the interview topics that I didn't get a chance to clarify during the interview?

Thank you very much for your attention

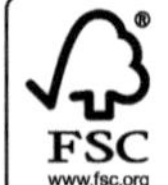

MIX
Papier aus verantwortungsvollen Quellen
Paper from responsible sources
FSC® C105338

Printed by Books on Demand GmbH, Norderstedt / Germany